AF753690

HIV/AIDS and Democratic Governance in South Africa

Illustrating the Impact on Electoral Processes

Edited by Per Strand and Kondwani Chirambo

The Governance and AIDS Programme staff:
Kondwani Chirambo, Programme Manager
Mary Caesar, Research Facilitator
Marietjie Myburg, Regional Media Coordinator
Bernard Likalimba, NGO Capacity-Building Coordinator
Vasanthie Naicker, Administrator
Shaila Gupta, Volunteer Researcher

Published by the Institute for Democracy in South Africa (IDASA)
Cnr Prinsloo and Visagie Streets
PO Box 56950
Arcadia 0007
Pretoria
South Africa
Tel: 27-12-3920500
Fax: 27-12-3202414/5
e-mails: kondwani@idasa.org.za; mary@idasa.org.za; marietjie@idasa.org.za
Website: www.idasa.org.za

© IDASA 2005
ISBN 1-919798-80-3 ISBN-13: 978-1-919798-80-6

First published 2005
Content edit by Per Strand and Kondwani Chirambo
Language edit by Moira Levy
Design and layout by Bronwen Müller
Cover by Mandy Darling, Magenta Media

This publication has been produced with the support of the Rockefeller Brothers Fund (RBF). The content of the publication is the sole responsibility of IDASA and can in no way be taken to reflect the views of the RBF.

Rockefeller Brothers Fund
Philanthropy for an Interdependent World

All rights reserved. No part of this publication may be reproduced or transmitted, in any form or by any means, without prior permission from the publishers.

Contents Page

Tables and Figures — Page

AUTHORS

Kondwani Chirambo is the manager of IDASA's Governance and AIDS Programme (GAP). He holds a Master of Arts (MA) degree in Mass Communications from the Faculty of Social Sciences, Centre for Mass Communication Research at the University of Leicester in the United Kingdom. He has written extensively on democratic processes in southern Africa, having worked on regional projects covering 11 countries. He has undertaken observations of electoral processes in eleven SADC countries in the past six years. Part of his election work has included evaluative research on electoral processes: Chirambo served as team leader of IDASA's research group that evaluated the impact of donor funding on electoral processes in Zambia in 2002-2003 on contract to five European governments. He has served as consultant also to the Electoral Institute of Southern Africa's (EISA's) evaluation of Zimbabwe's 2002 presidential elections (March, 2003) and to several SADC Parliamentary Forum election missions. Prior to joining IDASA-GAP in 2002 he served as head of the Democracy and Governance Programme at the Southern African Research and Documentation Centre (SARDC) in Harare, Zimbabwe. This AIDS and elections project was conceived and directed by him.

Per Strand holds a PhD in political science from Uppsala University in Sweden. His thesis – Decisions on Democracy: The Politics of Constitution-Making in South Africa 1990-1996 – seeks to explain how the compromise on the democratic constitution emerged through negotiations, brinkmanship and the recognition of mutual interests between the key parties. He has extensive experience of lecturing in Comparative Politics and Research Methodology at the departments of Political Studies at Uppsala University, the University of Cape Town and the University of the Western Cape. Strand is affiliated to the Centre for Social Science Research at the University of Cape Town where he does research on how the political responses to the HIV/AIDS epidemic in southern Africa impacts on the quality of democracy and good governance in the region. Strand is an IDASA research associate.

Consultant: **Khabele Matlosa** is the Senior Advisor (Director) in the Research Department at the Electoral Institute of Southern Africa (EISA). He holds a PhD in political economy from the University of the Western Cape, Cape Town, and an MA in development studies from the University of Leeds, UK. He has lectured extensively at undergraduate level on political development and governance in southern Africa at the National University of Lesotho (NUL), the University of the Western Cape and at post-graduate level on the Master of Policy Studies (MPS) programme of the Southern African Political Economy Series (SAPES) Trust based in Harare, Zimbabwe. Prior to joining EISA Dr Matlosa was the Director, Research and Policy Studies Faculty, at SAPES Trust. Dr Matlosa played a key role in the process of electoral reform in Lesotho that resulted in the change of the country's electoral system from the First-Past-The-Post electoral model to the new Mixed Member Proportional (MMP) electoral model in 2002.

Consultant: **Ann Elaine Strode** is senior lecturer at the School of Law, University of KwaZulu-Natal, Pietermaritzburg. She has served as special legal adviser to the National HIV/AIDS and STD Directorate and she is the regional director for Lawyers for Human Rights; was a member of the University of KwaZulu-Natal's HIV/AIDS vaccine and ethics research group and has consulted for international and donor agencies in various capacities. She recently completed a consultancy for IDASA's Governance and AIDS Project on Institutional Governance of the HIV/AIDS pandemic in South Africa. She holds An LLM, LLB and BA in religious studies and political science from the University of Natal.

Acknowledgements

Several key persons have been involved in one way or another in the process of undertaking this study. I wish to begin by expressing our profound gratitude to the Rockefeller Brother Fund (RBF) for taking the all important step of investing in this project. The field of AIDS and governance is relatively new and has but a handful of dedicated researchers and institutions investigating the broader implication of the pandemic for political, social and economic processes. It takes great courage and confidence to lend support to a hitherto untested project.

In the past two years the staff and associates of the Governance and Aids Programme (GAP), with the support of several key partnerships, have endeavoured to fulfil our vision firstly, to determine the manner and extent to which AIDS will impact on democratic consolidation, and secondly, to work with relevant governance institutions to develop appropriate responses in this regard. We owe the realisation of GAP as a regional project to the initial core support extended by the Ford Foundation in 2001 over a three-year period. I wish to thank our many respondents: the political parties involved in the study; the Independent Electoral Commission (IEC) of South Africa for making available its raw data and policy documents; Citizen Surveys for conducting our KwaZulu-Natal focus group discussions that form an important segment of this report; the People Living with HIV/AIDS and care givers who supported our project by attending the discussions; Derek Davids of the Afrobarometer project who provided important pointers on the use of public opinion data. The Electoral Institute of Southern Africa (EISA) seconded its Director of Research for the duration of the project. On behalf of the research team I wish to thank staff members of the IDASA-GAP for their commitment and resolve to see the project through. Mary Caesar, the research facilitator, Marietjtie Myburg, the regional media coordinator, Vasanthie Naicker, the project administrator and Shaila Gupta, the volunteer researcher from the US, dedicated valuable time to facilitate, organise, collate information and provide research backup. Above all, this project benefited greatly from the experience and wisdom of IDASA's Executive Director, Paul Graham, whose patience and confidence in the abilities of the programme staff resulted in this product. If we have failed to acknowledge others from whose valuable input we benefited, we do so with sincere apologies.

Kondwani Chirambo, Manager IDASA-GAP

Foreword

I often reflected upon the unprovided condition that the whole body of the people were in at the first coming of this calamity upon them, and how it was for want of timely entering into measures and managements, as well public as private, that all the confusions that followed were brought upon us, and that such a prodigious number of people sank in that disaster, which, if proper steps had been taken, might, Providence concurring, have been avoided, and which, if posterity think fit, they may take a caution and warning from.

Daniel Defoe wrote these words after a plague that killed 100 000 people in London in 1664 and 1665. His book, *A Journal of the Plague Years*, published in 1722 is worth reading. Looking back on the horror of those years, he numbers the dead, provides evidence of the impact of the plague on people's behaviour – panic, a descent into amorality by some and enormous courage by others – reflects on the desperate search for remedies in medicine, quackery, faith and superstition, and notes the very real commitment to the poor by the City of London and the more distant philanthropy of the Royal Court. His is not the only plague literature – Camus' *The Plague* provided important reading for those of us locked in by apartheid as it had originally reflected on the prison of occupied France – but its story of a plague-ridden city in which death provokes denial, escape, fatalism and courage resonates in our present time of plague.

Of course HIV/AIDS does not kill overnight. It is not a disease where, as one mediaeval poet wrote of the Black Death of 1347-1352 when between a quarter and a third of the European population died, "one could eat lunch with friends and have dinner with ancestors in paradise".

All the more reason then to take Daniel Defoe to heart. When IDASA made the argument in 2001 that led to the Ford Foundation supporting the establishment of a Governance and HIV/AIDS programme, it said:

AIDS is a wasting disease; it may be possible for the HIV negative to ignore the holocaust and even for the society to avoid the matter. This would be an ethical catastrophe that will haunt us for years to come. This is an opportunity to forge a society that values caring, that confronts the costs of healthcare, that orients itself around the needs of the poor and vulnerable, and that has learned to talk with and listen to the marginalised. These are not medical issues, they are issues of social reconstruction and governance.

In South Africa at least an estimated 28% of the adult population see HIV/AIDS as one of the most important problems facing this country "that the government should address". And it is common cause that civil society action, activism and altruism has flourished as the country comes to terms with levels of infection and now with rising numbers of deaths.

IDASA is not an HIV/AIDS or health services public benefit organisation. Our mandate expressed in our mission statement is promoting sustainable democracy in South Africa and elsewhere by building democratic institutions, educating citizens and advocating social justice. But, as Camus says in his novel, "This business is everybody's business". Hence the establishment of the Governance and AIDS Programme, which is interested both in fitting governance to meet the challenge of the disease and in understanding how the disease impacts on and potentially undermines democratic governance.

The research in this report is groundbreaking. It is an attempt to understand how HIV/AIDS can and does impact on electoral democracy using South Africa as a case; it thus has local relevance as well as a more general message to communicate. The work could not have been done without support from the Rockefeller Brothers Fund and GAP's initial funder, the Ford Foundation.

IDASA is committed to identifying and remedying those matters that threaten the capacity for democracy of the state and civil society. One of the most fundamental challenges – one which we dare not fail – is the challenge of HIV/AIDS. Treatment is giving us some additional time, but it has not removed the threat of death and disease either to individuals or to our democratic society.

For the first time this report confronts us with what the threat really is in the area of elections and thus the foundation of democratic governance. It recommends proper steps that need to be taken. Let some future Daniel Defoe not find us wanting.

Paul Graham, Executive Director

BACKGROUND AND OVERVIEW OF THE STUDY

The HIV/AIDS epidemic is a severe health crisis in South Africa and a challenge that goes far beyond the provision of medical treatment. The analytical framework of this report and the results we present show that the problematic impacts threaten to undermine South Africa's democratic project, while an effective response will require nothing less than the full mobilisation of the institutions, ideals and leaders that drive that democratic vision. Our investigation of the democratic governance aspects of the epidemic has naturally had the electoral process at its core.

This research project had the objective of investigating the probable impact of HIV/AIDS on electoral processes as a key facet of the democratisation process in Africa. The rationale is that democracy requires strong institutions and the full participation of citizens in political, social and economic life to be sustainable. However HIV/AIDS, as research has confirmed, is depleting the skills base in all developmental sectors and reducing the capacity of societies to be productive and secure the livelihoods of their citizens. Institutions might be weakened due to loss of skills and the sum effect would be to affect the quality of governance. Good governance, which has been equated to democratic governance by the United Nations Development Programme (UNDP) after all, is meant to deliver job opportunities, education and *long healthy lives for all citizens*, among other things.

The motivation to this study goes back to 2003 when IDASA's Governance and AIDS Programme (GAP), in collaboration with the UNDP HIV and Development Project for Sub-Saharan Africa, convened the Governance and AIDS Forum for Southern Africa in Cape Town, which brought together senior representatives from 12 Southern African Development Community (SADC) countries. Delegates came from the UNAIDS, UNDP, SADC Health Sector Coordinating Unit and SADC Parliamentary Forum, the Electoral Commission of SADC Countries, finance ministries and research institutions to discuss, analyse and seek solutions to the impact of HIV/AIDS on governance processes in Africa. One of the key concerns raised by the Electoral Management Bodies (EMBs) and research institutions was the possible impact of HIV/AIDS on key areas of the electoral process and the absence of coping mechanisms in most African countries.

In response to this IDASA-GAP, as the main convener, undertook this exploratory project as part of an Africa-wide intervention, beginning with South Africa. The following elements of the electoral process were examined:

- Electoral systems;
- Political institutions;
- Electoral management and administration;
- Voter participation.

We sought in the main to test hypotheses developed by IDASA and its associates, which interrogated the extent to which the AIDS pandemic would destabilise political processes, *if at all*.

We have asked – and sought to provide answers – to several key statements:

- That AIDS affects electoral systems differently;
- That the loss of skilled personnel in EMBs might impact on the efficiency with which elections are conducted;
- That HIV/AIDS is likely to shape public opinion with political and social ramifications;
- That People Living with HIV/AIDS (PLWHAs) and care givers will be marginalised from the electoral process (through stigma, discrimination and structural factors);
- That HIV/AIDS is reducing the pool of voters available to participate in elections and might have implications for political outcomes.

Our ambition with the research, therefore, was to assist EMBs and other state administrations in strengthening their future interventions in the area of electoral processes by gathering and analysing information that will support the formulation and implementation of effective responses to the HIV/AIDS pandemic. A comprehensive mapping exercise of South Africa has been undertaken with respect to the mortality of registered voter populations in the past five years and comparative analyses with selected Southern African countries in regard to the electoral systems have been conducted. HIV/AIDS policies of the Independent Electoral Commission (IEC), leading political parties and of the government have been analysed within the context of this topic. In addition, key interviews were undertaken with political parties as well as with registered voters who were infected with and affected by HIV/AIDS.

While the South African election in April 2004 was our most obvious empirical reference when we worked on the report, our ambition has been to formulate questions and explore methodologies, to discuss results and suggest recommendations that have a wider relevance so that democrats in other countries in the region and beyond can learn from South Africa's strengths and weaknesses. For these reasons we wish to highlight the following results and recommendations.

KEY FINDINGS

- **Voter mortality:** Our analyses of the deaths between 1999 and 2003 among voters registered on the voters' roll generate mortality profiles of different age cohorts of men and women that, on the whole, strengthen the argument that critical segments of the South African electorate are dying from AIDS. Increases in mortality over the four years for women 30-39 years old exceed 300 percent in some municipalities and 160 percent in the Limpopo province. Overall, between 1999 and 2003, 1 488 242 (almost 1.5 million) South African registered voters died of various causes. The heaviest casualties were between the age cohort 30-39 (29 percent of the deaths) and 40-49 (19 percent of the deaths). We argue that these problematic and abnormal mortality profiles in the electorate can to a large extent, if not wholly, be explained by AIDS. We base our argument on the strong correspondence between the profiles that our analysis generated and those that have been described by the expert demographers in the field of HIV/AIDS, as well as on our own statistical analyses. We note that it is fortunate that South Africa has citizen and voter registration systems that are directly compatible and therefore equipped to timeously update the voters' roll. In this regard the Independent Electoral Commission (IEC) of South Africa assures us that all dead voters were purged from the voters' roll before the 2004 elections; a development that should serve to allay fears or perceptions of "ghost voting".

- **Electoral Systems:** It is established that the Westminster electoral model, or First-Past-the Post (FPTP), is more vulnerable to HIV/AIDS than the Proportional Representation (PR) system. The FPTP has serious cost implications for sustainability. Preliminary evidence of by-elections generated by increased deaths and the cost of holding them is provided from three southern African countries to underline this fact. While South Africa uses the PR method at national level, it does operate a hybrid system (FPTP and PR) at local level and might yet endure the effects of the disease. Our analyses of the effect of AIDS on the PR list at national level and the local government system falls short of giving any specific conclusions on the impact of the disease, for lack of key information on the causes of deaths of MPs and councillors or any clear discernible pattern of mortality. Conversely, a pilot study by IDASA undertaken in 2003 in Zambia – which uses the FPTP electoral method – indicates that between 1964 and 1984 (the 20-year period before the advent of HIV/AIDS) a total of 46 by-elections were held and 14 of those were a result of death by illness and accidents combined. While over an 18-year period (from 1985, the year the first case of AIDS was documented in Zambia, to February 2003) 102 by-elections were held and 59 of those were due to death by disease. The majority of the 59 by-elections, a total of 39, were held between 1992 and February 2003, which coincidentally are the years in which the HIV/AIDS pandemic peaked in Zambia. While there might be no specific information on the nature of the illnesses that led to the deaths of representatives, trend analyses can be indicative of the influence of the pandemic. Using today's US dollar rates to the local kwacha currency, we find that Zambia has spent at least 200 000 US dollars on each by-election. Similarly, eight by-elections were held in Lesotho since the country modified the electoral model in 2002 from FPTP to a Mixed Member Proportional (MMP) system (which fuses FPTP with PR). Seven of these had been elected through the FPTP system and one through the PR system. The country has held about six by-elections already, each one costing about R1 million (about 161 300 US dollars). Three of the by-elections were caused by MPs' deaths. The seventh by-election is yet to be organised.
- **Power shifts:** We note that disease in general, and especially HIV/AIDS, will contribute to power shifts in countries operating the FPTP electoral model. The effect of illness, combined with vacancies generated by expulsions, resignations or floor-crossing by members, has compelled Zimbabwe to hold 13 (+1) by-elections since the 2000 legislative polls. Eight of the by-elections arose because parliamentary representatives had died prematurely of "illness".

The sum effect is that the opposition parties have lost the majority of the by-elections, partly perhaps due to their inability to compete perpetually with a well-resourced ruling party. As South Africa has been engaged in debates over electoral reform in the recent past, it is imperative that the implications of electoral reform in this direction are critically examined, given the experience of neighbouring countries.

- **Electoral management and administration:** Our analyses of the internal policy of the Independent Electoral Commission (IEC) of South Africa and of existing studies on the impact of HIV/AIDS on parastatal/state institutional skills bases suggest that the IEC, which relies on public service workers for support during elections, is vulnerable to the pandemic's effects that might compromise its institutional capacities. This vulnerability is aggravated by the fact that most temporary staff are from the public service, particularly the teaching profession, which is one of the hardest hit by the HIV/AIDS pandemic. As the conduct of elections requires experienced staff, the vulnerability of support personnel to the disease is likely to reduce the IEC's ability to rely on them to bring their accumulated experience and skills to bear on future elections. And with the following age structure in its permanent staff – four staff members aged 18-24 years, 178 staff 25-49 years and 28 staff 50-60 years – the IEC is vulnerable to the much higher HIV prevalence and effects of AIDS among young and middle-aged adults.
- **Special vote:** It is acknowledged that the "special vote" is a useful institutional arrangement to ensure, as far as possible, that people are not disenfranchised by being ill, disabled or pregnant or by virtue of attending to business or educational trips abroad. The mere fact that it exists and was delivered to more than 650 000 voters in the last election is a powerful indication of the commitment of the South African authorities to making democratic participation through the vote as inclusive as possible. However there is a need to state categorically to the public whether people suffering from debilitating or chronic illnesses qualify for this facility. We do find for instance that some people living with HIV/AIDS who might wish to have access to the special vote lack sufficient information on whether they are eligible or not. This is likely to have implications for participation by people who are infected with diseases such as HIV/AIDS that are accompanied by stigma and discrimination.
- **Political parties:** Of the leading political parties in South Africa, the ANC and Inkatha Freedom Party (IFP) acknowledge that HIV/AIDS has put some strain on their party structures by creating an increased need to replace cadres who have succumbed to illness or who have died. Although no severe functional defects have arisen in the party structures, the loss of seniority and experience nevertheless is reported to have reduced parties' capacities and "intellectual memory" somewhat. A more direct impact is acknowledged by a religious-based party, the African Christian Democratic Party (ACDP), which says that political leaders who are also church ministers have had to commit increasing amounts of time to officiate at funerals in their respective congregations. This affected negatively their ability to participate in weekend campaign meetings for the party in the run-up to the 2004 elections.

- **Public opinion:** More detailed analyses of the Afrobarometer public opinion data from southern African countries (including South Africa) suggest an increase generally in public awareness of HIV/AIDS as a political and social problem. There is, however, no basis to argue that HIV/AIDS is shaping public opinion in a consistent fashion across the southern African region. South Africa is an exception though as statistical patterns indicate that people who suffer personal loss are more likely to prioritise HIV/AIDS in their demands on government interventions. The survey from 2002 does not, however, suggest that people affected by HIV/AIDS would change their choice of political party as a result of this disaffection.
- **Stigma and discrimination** resonated as the most dominant determinants for lack of participation in elections by PLWHAs and care givers. Focus group discussions held in urban and rural areas of KwaZulu-Natal with PLWHAs and care givers who were *all registered voters* for the 2004 election yielded seemingly well-founded fears that communities would ostracise or marginalise those infected and affected further if they exposed themselves to the major public events. The respondents' opinions correlate with the findings of studies on stigma and discrimination, particularly South Africa's Department of Health study of 2002, that HIV/AIDS remains a taboo among some South African communities, especially in the rural enclaves. The sense of stigma, it seems, would be strongest among people who are symptomatic; respondents argued that most members of the communities would not stand in the same queue with someone with visible signs of disease, for example body rashes or sores. Based on these discussions we concluded that people who have visible signs of illness from HIV/AIDS, and those who have publicly declared their status, are more likely to eschew from public voting, particularly if they are located in a rural area. There is nothing to suggest in the main that PLWHAs have lost the will to participate in political life. Quite the contrary: the majority of respondents expressed a desire to participate, but were constrained by attitudinal and structural factors. These results are not representative of the opinions of all PLWHAs as only 68 people participated in the focus groups, but they are indicative of such attitudes and might have external validity.

KEY RECOMMENDATIONS

The concept *democratic governance* carries much normative weight and can potentially be a powerful advocacy tool for a strong political response against the epidemic. As with all such concepts, however, it runs a risk of becoming meaningless, a mere rhetorical phrase, if it is not used in a critical and politically forthright analytical framework that recognises the many previous governance failures on the continent.

INSTITUTIONAL/STRUCTURAL REFORM

- Given that an electoral system is the instrument for translating votes cast in an election into seats in legislative assemblies for elected representatives, the impact of HIV/AIDS on the system has a direct bearing on the functioning of the two most important representative institutions, parliament and local government authorities. Thus one of the most important ways in which the political ramifications of HIV/AIDS on elections can be unveiled by both the academic and policy communities is to discover the direct and/or indirect impact of the epidemic on electoral systems as part of the broader electoral reform agenda.
- As SADC countries embark upon electoral reforms, issues around HIV/AIDS should be taken on board in the determination of the appropriate electoral systems to be adopted. By all indications, both the financial and political costs of the HIV/AIDS pandemic are more onerous in countries that operate the FTPT electoral system than those that operate the PR system. In this regard South Africa is better off retaining its PR model at the national level.
- Currently legislation does not allow for a special vote for people who are unable to travel to polling stations during local government elections. This is a significant omission which might effectively mean that many people infected with HIV or affected by the epidemic will be disenfranchised during local government elections. It is recommended that the IEC should appeal to the Justice Portfolio Committee in parliament that the Local Government Municipal Electoral Act, No 24 of 2000 be amended to create a right to special votes in local government elections.
- The IEC should finalise the current skills succession plan to ensure that it will have sufficient skilled staff in strategic positions and that HIV/AIDS focal point persons are appointed in all offices or that certain staff take responsibility for HIV/AIDS activities. Such tasks should be part of their formal job descriptions.
- Political parties should consider institutionalising a strong response against the epidemic within its own party structures and membership. The need for democratic governance on HIV/AIDS does not only apply to governments and states, but also to the political parties that, through their actions, set the norms for what should be an effective government policy and a humane and tolerant attitude in society.

PUBLIC OPINION AND PARTICIPATION

- The urgency with which HIV/AIDS is addressed through policy by governments and the emphasis it is given by international agencies is not clearly reflected in public perceptions as these are captured in the most current (from 2002) and comprehensive opinion surveys from sub-Saharan Africa. It is not clear yet how this should be understood and more research is needed. The fact that no obvious political momentum is stirred by issues relating to HIV/AIDS among the electorates in the region does not, however, necessarily imply a lack of concern. Politicians should engage communities to mobilise a political awareness that can be channelled constructively as part of an overall response to the epidemic.

- Our results from testing the problematic hypothesis that those directly infected with or affected by the epidemic are more likely not to participate in the electoral process were confirmed, with two exceptions. The lack of data at appropriate levels of analysis, however, generates results that are inherently unstable and thus offer no solid base for political action. Governments and electoral commissions in southern Africa are called upon to assist with the necessary data to enable research with a regional scope that can produce more authoritative results.
- Our analysis of the mortality profiles among the South African electorate, on the basis of data from the voters' roll, generated information that amounts to the veritable "smoking gun" of AIDS-related mortality. These results should mobilise additional energy for the political response to the epidemic at local, provincial and national levels of government. The information should further be discussed by local communities, with local authorities, to stem an increase in deaths that in some places is alarmingly high.

STRATEGIC INTERVENTIONS

- **Formation of bi-partisan coalitions:** It is recommended that there be greater involvement of political leaders – Members of Parliament and councillors in particular – in public education campaigns to reduce stigma and discrimination, possibly one of the most compelling factors that could impact on voter turnout and registration. This might require the establishment of a strategic bi-partisan extra-parliamentary body that involves all the elected national representatives. Tanzania, for instance, has established the Tanzania Parliamentarians AIDS Coalition (TAPAC) the membership of which is open to former and serving MPs from all parties. As TAPAC is an NGO and, therefore, not an integral part of the parliamentary system, it has served to empower MPs, enabled interaction with constituencies and AIDS bodies and continued to improve their advocacy role to enable strong leadership at parliamentary level, while maintaining HIV/AIDS on the agenda in parliamentary committees. As nearly all MPs are members of TAPAC, this setup provides a good example of a practical way of depoliticising HIV/AIDS, while dealing with issues such as stigma and discrimination.
- **Use of traditional governance systems:** It is further recommended that greater emphasis be placed by state and non-state actors in the area of HIV/AIDS on empowering traditional leaders to assist in redressing the problems of stigma and discrimination in rural enclaves to allow for greater participation of PLWHAs in political, social and economic life. The role of

traditional leaders in public education and their influence thereof is underlined by respondents in this study who view them as some of the key change agents to deal with stigma and discrimination in their respective communities. The potential of traditional governance systems to enhance service delivery and to ensure that rural populations are not marginalised from development was also underlined and acknowledged by the Africa Development Forum (ADF) 1V, co-hosted in Addis Ababa, Ethiopia, by the Economic Commission for Africa, the African Union and the African Development Bank in October 2004. Respondents in this study also confirm the critical role played by traditional leaders in sensitising communities on various issues. The use of kingships, councillors and religious leaders through community radio networks and public forums in this regard is highly recommended owing to the high degree of esteem they seem to command, particularly in rural settings.

- **HIV/AIDS in voter and civic education:** It is imperative that the IEC builds HIV/AIDS awareness into its voter education programmes to help reduce the extent of HIV/AIDS stigma and discrimination inherent in communities. Establishing linkages with HIV/AIDS service providers and civic education groups should help develop context specific approaches to deal with misconceptions about HIV/AIDS and possibly improve or sustain high participation levels. Apart from emphasising all aspects of HIV/AIDS, including prevention, treatment and nutrition, there should be emphasis on the human/political rights of all individuals in the IEC's and civic groups' public communication programmes.
- **General comment:** We note that South Africa has launched possibly the largest treatment programme in the world. Although the mechanics of it are yet to be lubricated, we see a potential in this programme for contributing significantly to the efforts to reduce HIV/AIDS-related stigma and discrimination. The sooner the pandemic is seen less as "a death sentence" than a chronic illness, the better for the communities that constantly ostracise PLWHAs for fear of contagion.

GOVERNMENT AND PUBLIC REACTION TO THE IDASA STUDY

When this study was disseminated to the public on 25 November, 2004, it generated wide media coverage and much intellectual debate beyond the borders of South Africa and Africa in general. We also, in this regard, take note of the official response of the Government of the Republic of South Africa to the study, which in many ways, appears balanced in framing appreciation for the recommendations and in applying more critical comment. The full text of the government response is in Appendix D of this book.

Part 1

Democratic Governance in the Context of the HIV & AIDS Epidemic

While much analytical attention has been spent on exploring how electoral systems differ in their construction and in terms of what democratic principles they entrench, little if any attention has been given to how sensitive they are to the effects of an epidemic such as HIV/AIDS.

Chapter 1

Introduction

South Africa staged its third national elections in April 2004 with a level of confidence found only in established democracies. Although political violence in the KwaZulu-Natal province unfortunately caused some casualties in the run-up to the elections and there were some instances of alleged irregularities, few would have thought, in the midst of the violence and uncertainties of the historic 1994 elections, that such efficiency and legitimacy would characterise the polls only ten years hence. The same can be said for the many substantial advances that have been made to improve basic living conditions and place the South African national economy on a much more solid footing. But on the crucial question of fighting the HIV/AIDS epidemic there are few real advances to record. While it is safe to say that the reasons for this failure are many, only some of which can be laid at the government's door, it is not the aim of this report to further explore the strengths and weaknesses of South Africa's political response to the epidemic – otherwise a common debate in academia and media. Our analysis is aimed instead at deepening our understanding of how the epidemic might impact on the democratic process as such. Instead of asking what political dynamics can explain a particularly problematic epidemic, we turn the question around and ask how the epidemic will impact on South Africa's democratic politics. In the course of our research one problematic paradox has become clear to us: while South Africa has made considerable advances in terms of development and the consolidation of democracy in the past ten years, its belated efforts to respond effectively to the HIV/AIDS epidemic might turn those advances into Pyrrhic victories in that the epidemic threatens to undo many of the positive developments that have been accomplished since 1994.

The main message from this research is that the legitimacy and effectiveness of the South African democracy and its electoral processes risk being undermined by the HIV/AIDS epidemic. Our central general argument is that while civil society organisations and the elected political representatives need to counter this threat by generating the necessary political will and commitment through the democratic process, this will be possible only once we better understand how and why the logic to democratic politics can hinder such a mobilisation of resources. Although our research in this report addresses only one aspect of the democratic process – the electoral process – we hope that it nevertheless will inform and inspire academics, activists and elected legislators alike in a public debate through which we can jointly formulate the strategies that will prove successful in halting the epidemic that ravages through the societies in southern Africa.

1.1 SETTING THE RESEARCH AGENDA

The HIV epidemic is one of the most significant public health threats to South Africa. By its very nature, however, it is not just a public health problem, but one that has wide-ranging socioeconomic implications for affected societies. Furthermore it has become increasingly clear that there is a link between the HIV/AIDS epidemic and good governance; a common and worrying argument is that an uncontrolled HIV epidemic poses a threat to democracy. This report is an empirical investigation into this question with the ambition to learn more about the link between the epidemic and governance and to test some more or less alarming arguments about the impact of the epidemic on the sustainability of democracy.

The report focuses on one of the quintessential aspects of and processes within any democracy: the electoral process. The general rationale for this choice of focus is that if the epidemic does have an impact it is more likely to be felt when the democratic process hinges on the active participation of the majority of citizens. And the relative importance of addressing the problem will increase if the epidemic impacts on the legitimacy and effectiveness of as central an institution as the democratic legislatures. This report therefore examines the electoral process and poses the question: *What impact did the HIV/AIDS epidemic have on the electoral process leading up to the 2004 national and provincial elections in South Africa?*

Elections are one of the cornerstones of democracy. They are the institutional mechanism through which citizens choose their national, provincial and local political representatives. They enable citizens to participate in re-electing or replacing political leaders, thus holding politicians and parties accountable for their performance while in office. While elections in a political system are not sufficient for calling it a democracy, the absence of elections in any political regime is sufficient for calling it an authoritarian system of one kind or another. However, given the experience of racially exclusive elections in apartheid South Africa, it is necessary to state that all adult citizens must have the right to partake on an equal basis. The South African Constitutional Court has emphasised the importance of voting in uniting a heterogeneous population with a history of internal conflict:

> *The achievement of the franchise has historically been important ... for the acquisition of the right of full and effective citizenship by all South Africans regardless of race... The vote of each and every citizen is a badge of dignity and personhood... In a country of great disparities of wealth and power it declares that whoever we are, whether rich or poor, exalted or disgraced, we all belong to the same democratic South African nation (August and Another v Electoral Commission and Others at para. 17).*

Given the centrality of the electoral process to any democracy, and its critical role in consolidating a unified democratic society in South Africa, there is obviously a need to correctly understand any development that poses a threat to its political legitimacy and institutional effectiveness. A number of contributions to an emerging international social science literature on the impact of HIV/AIDS on civil and political society formulate some of the central arguments and hypotheses that we will try to test in this report. However, to the best of our knowledge, there is no contribution that explicitly, through systematic empirical research, explores what impact the epidemic might have on electoral processes. For these and other reasons (see section 1.3 on methodological concerns below) the research that we present here should be regarded as explorative in that it has few or no previous empirical findings to relate to and little in terms of specialised and tested methodological instruments to apply. The report will hopefully, therefore, apart from presenting some substantial research results, inform other similar research projects on what methods and avenues of investigation might prove effective and fruitful.

To provide additional focus to our analysis, the report researches the following four key aspects of the 2004 South African elections:

- The electoral systems that establish the rules for elections;
- Institutions established to manage the elections (ie the Independent Electoral Commission);
- Political institutions (the parties contesting the elections); and
- The level of voter participation in the elections.

The broad approach that these four aspects signify is indicative of the explorative nature of this research project. While this approach enables us to comment on a number of aspects related to the research question, we have not been able to explore any of them in depth to the extent they deserve. Our more general discussions in Part One of the report (chapters 1-3) seeks to provide the necessary analytical context for our discussion by presenting key epidemiological data, analytical concepts and central hypotheses. In Part Two of the report (chapters 4-6) we apply these discussions to the three institutional aspects that were presented above – electoral systems, the independent electoral commission and the political parties. In Part Three (chapters 7-10), finally, we explore the impact on voter participation.

1.2 OBJECTIVES OF THE RESEARCH PROJECT

The following broader objectives of our research have provided guidance throughout the research process and in formulating the analytical narrative in the report:

- To generate evidence-based information as an advocacy tool to facilitate concerted action from the government and the state, particularly from those institutions that are involved directly in the electoral processes and thereby influence law and policy;
- To develop the debate and discussion on possible solutions and interventions that will assist government and specifically electoral institutions in mitigating the impact of the epidemic on democratic consolidation, thus averting possible electoral conflict;
- To raise the awareness about the links between the epidemic and democratic governance among the public in general and among activists and policymakers in particular; and
- To help facilitate improved communication and a constructive exchange of research ideas between scholars across academic disciplines who are all doing research on HIV/AIDS.

It is our hope that, through different channels of influence, the report will assist in the formulation of a National HIV/AIDS Strategy that will prevent new HIV infections, provide greater access to care, treatment and support, as well as mitigate the adverse social, political and economic effects of the epidemic on the prospects for sustaining and deepening the South African democracy. To reach as broad a readership as possible, the report does not assume much knowledge in the reader about the issues discussed and therefore provides considerable background information. As a consequence, not all chapters will be equally relevant to some readers with particular expertise. But this is arguably preferable to excluding readers along the way.

1.3 THE HIV/AIDS EPIDEMIC AND THE ELECTORAL PROCESS

UNAIDS, the United Nations body that coordinates the UN and other global efforts in fighting the epidemic, estimates that 5.3 million, or between 4.5 and 6.2 million, South Africans of all ages were infected with HIV at the end of 2003, the majority of whom are women. This places South Africa at the top of the unenviable list of countries in terms of absolute numbers of infected residents, with India a close second at 5.1 million, or between 2.5 and 8.5 million (UNAIDS, 2004).

With a start to the epidemic in the early 1990s, South Africa has only more recently entered the phase when its devastating effects will become increasingly clear and painful in terms of a sharp increase in AIDS-related morbidity and mortality. That is unless a quick and extensive treatment campaign can effectively halt this tragic development. The nature, extent and variations of the epidemic in South Africa are presented and discussed in chapter two.

Issues relating to HIV/AIDS have been steeped in politics ever since what would later be named "AIDS" was first brought to the world's attention with the discovery of unusual cancers among members of San Francisco's gay community in the early 1980s (Epstein, 1996; Shilts, 1987).

It was ignorance and prejudice that first singled out gay men as the only group at risk of infection and it took much political activism to raise general awareness and fight the stigma that is attached to sexually transferable deceases, especially one that at first was thought to originate somehow in homosexuality. The allocation of public resources to research, care and treatment was also an inherently political issue once the epidemic had moved beyond the gay community to establish a grip in the majority "mainstream" heterosexual population. But it is, arguably, only recently, and then only in some particularly affected developing countries, that the epidemic has entered the realm of electoral politics. It is in countries such as those in southern Africa, where prevalence levels in some instances surpass 30% and life-expectancy has dropped significantly, that the epidemic can be suspected to have an impact on the legitimacy, effectiveness and outcomes of electoral processes.

It is in these contexts, where the epidemic is such a blatant threat to the economic and institutional prerequisites for the consolidation of democracy, that the social and political dimensions of the epidemic should be analysed with some urgency to better understand how it impacts on the prospects for democracy and development. What can be learned from fighting the epidemic in Southern Africa can hopefully prevent similar prevalence levels from ever occurring elsewhere. The links between HIV/AIDS and democracy are discussed in chapter three of the report, with "democratic governance" as the central concept.

1.3.1 ELECTORAL SYSTEM

The electoral system in a democracy is the crucial institutional device through which opinions among the electorate are translated into seats and power in legislatures. While much analytical attention has been spent on exploring how electoral systems differ in their construction and in terms of what democratic principles they entrench, little if any attention has been given to how sensitive they are to the effects of an epidemic such as HIV/AIDS. In chapter four we will present the South African electoral system and explore its relative weaknesses and strengths in the face of the epidemic with alternative electoral systems in southern Africa as points of comparison.

1.3.2 ELECTORAL COMMISSIONS

Since elections settle disputes about power they always will be susceptible to fraud. All democracies have therefore institutionalised procedures of one form or another that seek to ensure that elections are truly "free and fair". In the recently democratised countries in southern Africa, such Electoral Management Bodies (EMBs) are vital for accrediting the election result with the stamp of approval that the elected regime needs to win national and international legitimacy. To successfully carry out its mandate, an EMB needs both qualified and experienced staff as well as accurate demographic statistics to feed into the national voters' roll. Where the HIV/AIDS epidemic reduces the availability of such appropriately qualified staff and where increased mortality is not accurately reflected in the voters' roll, the risk of electoral fraud increases manifold. Although the South African democracy, and its Independent Electoral Commission, is better resourced than those in neighbouring countries there is no basis for assuming that it is immune to the problematic effects of the epidemic, hence our analysis of the South African IEC in chapter five.

1.3.3 POLITICAL PARTIES

Given the overwhelmingly representative nature of democracy in the world today, the political parties that contest elections to win seats in legislative assemblies are of course absolutely essential for the democratic process. While Members of Parliament (MPs) win personal mandates from electoral constituencies in countries like Botswana and Zambia, these nevertheless co-ordinate their parliamentary work under direction from their respective political parties. Under the alternative electoral system, where voters can vote only for parties and not individual MPs, as in South Africa and Namibia, the parties are all the more important for the electoral process and the legislative work in parliament. Where the HIV/AIDS epidemic undermines parties' capacity to campaign in elections and to effectively represent its voters during parliamentary sessions – through the loss of leaders, MPs and active members to AIDS-related illnesses and death – parties will be less representative of the electorate and less effective in shaping legislation in accordance with the mandate they have been given by their voters.

To what extent the epidemic can be said to have impacted negatively on the South African parties in their 2004 election campaigns, and how the parties respond to the epidemic more generally, is discussed in chapter six of the report.

1.3.4 VOTER PARTICIPATION

A democratic system might have an elaborate constitution and strong institutions to uphold its letter and spirit, but without vibrant participation from individuals and organisations in civil society, democracy, arguably, becomes an empty ritual for procedural power games between contending elites, far removed from the ideal of participatory democracy. There are of course different normative views on how much popular participation is ideal for democracy and how institutional arrangements should be shaped so as to provide opportunities and incentives for participation throughout the parliamentary process, but among democrats of all persuasions there should be little room for disagreement about the desirability of a high electoral turnout. Academics and politicians alike therefore argue about the causes of a troubling international trend of decreasing turnout in democratic elections and different hypotheses are suggested for why increasing numbers of people who can vote choose not to do so. The HIV/AIDS epidemic suggests the reverse logic to explain non-participation in elections: people who want to cast their votes are unable to do so due to illnesses and/or burdens imposed on them by the epidemic. Chapter seven in the report will introduce our analysis of voter participation by exploring what basis there is in the data from public opinion surveys across southern Africa to argue that the epidemic has an effect on people's willingness and/or ability to take active part in political life. We shall use this data also to describe how people's opinions differ on issues related to HIV/AIDS and explore how these differences can be understood. In chapter eight we present an analysis based on electoral data from the IEC, demographic data from

StatisticsSA and epidemiological data from various sources to describe not only how the actual numbers of registered voters vary, but also how those numbers relate to estimates of what is the complete Voting Age Population (VAP) in South Africa. By relating these data to various estimates of the epidemic in South Africa we explore what basis there is for arguing that voter participation was hampered by the direct and indirect effects of the epidemic.

Chapter nine presents a unique set of information from the voters' roll in an analysis of the "mortality profiles" of the South African electorate. In chapter ten we juxtapose the statistical analyses in chapters 7-9 with the voices of individual South Africans to try to contextualise our statistical findings in the human stories and wise reflections by a number of potential voters who are either infected with or directly affected by the epidemic. In chapter eleven, finally, we present our general conclusions and specific recommendations.

1.4 METHODOLOGICAL CONCERNS

It was mentioned above that our research on the impact of the HIV/AIDS epidemic on the electoral process in South Africa should be seen as explorative as there is no similar previous research on which to draw and no specific and tested methodological instrument to apply. In taking up this challenge we used four key methodological approaches. In our literature review we consulted national as well as international titles from academic, activist and official discourses on governance and the epidemic. We analysed a number of key documents, including the legal and constitutional frameworks governing the electoral process and central epidemiological reports[1], and we also gathered specific information from the South African parliament and the various central election manifestos from the parliamentary parties as well as from policy declarations by the IEC. To probe the policies and practices of some of the political parties we conducted semi-structured interviews with their respective HIV/AIDS spokespersons. The same interview format was used to attain valuable information from a few centrally placed senior officials of the IEC. Most of these interviews were recorded. The party representatives who so wished have had a chance to edit our write-up of those interviews to ensure that they had not been misunderstood. Our analysis of quantitative data – that is, information in the form of numbers – always starts with mere descriptions of how frequencies vary across different provinces, different groups in the population or whatever the case might be, but we then take one step further in our statistical analysis by exploring to what extent there are "patterns" in the data by doing correlation analyses. The main purpose of these is to establish if there is a statistical connection between factors A and B, for example if it is true that a person who is very busy with providing home-based care is less likely to be politically active in civil society.

In one instance we also explore the basis for a causal argument through a slightly more advanced regression analysis. Our narrative in these parts of the report will not assume any knowledge in statistics or exclude any reader who is uncomfortable with numbers. Finally, through six focus group discussions, we were privileged to get into direct contact with up to 68 people who were either People Living with HIV/AIDS (PLWHAs) and/or care givers who shared their personal and immediate experiences with us of political and social activity in general and of the April elections in particular. These six discussions were held in three rural and three urban centres in KwaZulu-Natal. In addition to these four methodologies we opened our research process to critical scrutiny through a stakeholder dialogue in early April 2004 that brought together electoral officials, political party representatives, experts from the UNDP and UNAIDS, international and local research agencies, donor agencies and media representatives. Representatives of key government ministries also were invited.

Having stated the four main methodologies, the following limitations should be brought to the reader's attention when considering our report. The depth, strength and relevance of our analyses in Parts Two and Three of the report are, obviously, dependent on the amount and quality of the empirical data that was available to us. To begin with, there is no reliable information on the precise reason for the death of an MP or local councillor or the vacancy due to illness of a parliamentary seat and such information should not be available without the consent of the individual or his/her surviving family. Discussions about the link between the sustainability of electoral systems and parliaments on the one hand, and the impact of the HIV/AIDS epidemic on the other, should therefore be read with caution. Does this lack of analytical precision mean that this type of research is futile? Certainly not. As long as the research is transparent about the need to extrapolate the impact of AIDS from basic information – and makes explicit the uncertainties that result from this – as well as follows the established ethical rules for social science research in other respects (Baylies and Bujra, 1997) it is imperative that we seek to make visible the problematic effects that otherwise would undermine the democratic process while everyone was looking the other way.

Our statistical analyses in chapters seven to nine also need some introductory comments. When using the Afrobarometer surveys in chapter seven for analysing the effects of the epidemic on people's opinions and on whether they are engaged in activities in civil society, we have to work with questions that are proxies for HIV and/or AIDS since direct questions on the HIV status of the respondent or of those in his/her care would be highly unreliable. Some of the questions we work with in that chapter therefore capture also other illnesses and conditions than those caused by AIDS. A problem with our statistical analyses of voter participation on the basis of electoral data from the IEC in chapter eight is that we can work only at the level of the nine provinces. That is, in testing whether, for instance, it is the case that registration was lower in provinces with higher estimates of HIV prevalence we were able to work only with nine cases (N=9). Statistical correlation analysis should be done ideally on a larger number of cases than that, since the results become somewhat less reliable and more difficult to interpret with so few cases. This does not mean that the analyses generate invalid results, but that they need to be interpreted with some caution. The same applies for the correlation analyses we do in the subsequent chapter nine on the information from the voters' roll. It should be noted further that since the analyses in chapters eight and nine are done on all nine cases the indication of statistical significance for the correlation coefficients become largely irrelevant. The opposite is the case in chapter seven where we analyse a sample that is representative of the whole population.[2] These limitations in the data we have had to work with imply that the statistical analyses we present are rather blunt methodological instruments for testing the link between the epidemic and non-participation in the election. This will be reflected in how we formulate our conclusions. On the basis of correlation analysis we can say whether there are any grounds for making the general argument that the epidemic has something to do with the level of non-participation on the level of the provinces. If such correlations can be established there are good reasons for exploring the issue in further depth also through other methodologies. One such attempt is made in this report in our commissioning of six focus group interviews with people who are infected with HIV or in other ways directly affected by the consequences of AIDS. The methodology used in focus group discussions can, with the help of special computer software, be analysed with a high degree of systematic rigour that can generate results with some degree of representivity if participants were chosen on correct grounds. Our usage of the material from the focus groups interviews was however less ambitious than that.

We use it here mainly to explore further some of the results that were indicated by our statistical analysis. That is, given what we learned from analysing electoral and epidemiological data through statistical means, we wished to put questions directly to the people most concerned to see if they could shed further light on the possible links between the epidemic and questions relating to political participation more generally and in the recent election more specifically. In brief we use the material from the focus groups with an explorative ambition, with an urge to learn more from the life stories and personal reflections of people who otherwise are seldom listened to.

When we discuss and perhaps make demands on certain policies from a democratic government to combat HIV/AIDS we need to remember that our most basic and principled expectation of democracy as a political system cannot be that it has particular foresight about future problems or that it is especially effective in dealing with them, but that it is responsive to citizens' demands as their needs change over time.

Chapter 2

The HIV/AIDS Epidemic in South Africa

2.1 INTRODUCTION

To contextualise our analysis of how the HIV/AIDS epidemic impacted on the 2004 elections we need to present and discuss the most relevant and current epidemiological data. In doing this, however, we shall seek to go beyond the mere reporting of statistical estimates and also discuss how they were arrived at and why they differ. We shall widen the discussion further to include demographic and developmental statistics since these are vital for understanding the contextual complexity that a governance perspective implies for the epidemic. Before we review and comment on the data in some detail, however, we need to take a step back and reflect on some aspects of what the nature of the epidemic implies for the political realm of a democracy in general and electoral outcomes in South Africa in particular.

2.1.1 DEMOCRACY AND EPIDEMICS

An initial anecdotal observation effectively brings home the main argument in this section that, by definition, epidemics are a threat to democracy. In his analysis of political implication of HIV/AIDS in Africa, Jeremy Youde notes that at an election rally in Kenya in 1997 a nurse was seen holding a placard with the message "*Don't worry about elections. All the voters will be dead!*" (Youde, forthcoming: 3). Indeed the connection between democracy and the epidemic/pandemic can be traced back to common etymological roots. In the word democracy, the Greek word *demos* represents the group of people who take collectively binding decisions. In the words epidemic and pandemic (that is, an epidemic that has spread across countries), *demos* represents the group of people who, in the case of HIV, are infected with a deadly virus. In southern Africa, more so than in any other part of the world, these two groups of people overlap to an alarming degree.

The Kenyan nurse was right: if left alone to ravage through the population, HIV/AIDS would reduce democracy to an exclusive business for the few who can still stand up.

An infectious disease is defined as an epidemic once infection rates increase rapidly in a population, as HIV prevalence did in South Africa throughout the 1990s, from below 1% in 1990 to just under 25% in 1998 (Whiteside and Sunter 2000). Because of the nature of the epidemic, however, it would be unrealistic to expect broad-based popular demands for a strong political response at an early stage in the epidemic. Figure 1 on the next page depicts the logic of the epidemic and its effects in three consecutive S-shaped curves – the three "waves" of the epidemic. In the first stages of the epidemic the virus spreads in a population by stealth, exploiting prejudice and denial to the fullest.

It is only after some time, ranging between four to eight years depending on the person's general health in other regards, that the direct medical effects of the virus will start to show in those who were first infected. At that point (T1) the

Figure 1. Epidemic curves, HIV, AIDS and impact

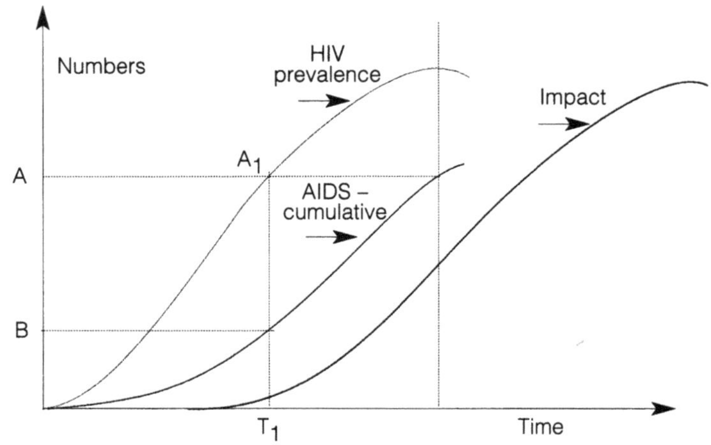

number of those who display opportunistic diseases due to a low CD4 count (B) is dwarfed by an "invincible" but much higher number of HIV-positive people (A). At this relatively early stage of the epidemic there is as yet little impact from the epidemic on society more generally.

But, if little is done to prevent further infections and treat those who are ill in the next few years, the direct and indirect costs of the epidemic will increase dramatically. At some stage in the future (T2) the epidemic might start to decline, but even at this stage the detrimental effects of the epidemic on society more generally will still increase for some time because of how families, communities, corporations and state bureaucracies have not yet compensated for the losses made in terms of personal grief and viability of households, social capital, labour resources and human skills (Whiteside and Barnett, 2002).

But we can also discuss figure 1 in a way that relates to the logic of democracy, in particular in a context where a new democratic regime has committed itself to fighting various manifestations of poverty and injustice, as is the case in South Africa. Given that many pressing demands for costly state interventions to reduce poverty are made on such a government, it will take great leadership from all actors in the political establishment also to prioritise the fight against HIV while prevalence is still at a relatively low level and no direct effects of the epidemic can be seen yet. At this early stage there will be little awareness among the population at large of what is happening and what effective prevention would imply for individual behaviour. In other words the voters in general do not see the need for state intervention and would not necessarily accept the remedies. In brief, at this early stage, a costly and demanding policy of prevention is not how the governing party ensures its re-election in the next election. In the short term (until the next election) the political incentives are rather in favour of downplaying the crisis. These incentives are, however, likely to shift in favour of strong political action once the explicit effects of the epidemic are felt in terms of AIDS sickness and death.

The realisation by increasing numbers of voters that an epidemic is upon them might translate into political demands for prevention and treatment. In responding to these demands the political establishment now faces a much bigger problem that will be much more difficult and costly to address than it would have been earlier in the epidemic when they had the necessary information to take action, but lacked the political incentive to do so.

The later in the process that the government finally responds, the bigger the task will be to combat the epidemic. Even once successful interventions have started to reduce the scale of the epidemic, the government will still face more long-term and structural effects of the epidemic for a long time to come, reducing its possibilities to address other poverty-related issues. Indeed if we today introduced a vaccine against AIDS-related deceases and effectively stopped all further infections of the virus, society would still battle with the effects of the epidemic for another 40 years (Shisana 2002).

In brief, the sooner in the epidemiological cycle the government acts the better. But an early response will be possible only if the government commits itself to carrying the political costs for doing so, ultimately the risk of loosing power for pushing an unpopular policy. This political risk will be reduced or eliminated altogether if the major parties agree to depoliticise the issue by forming a broad policy accord on HIV/AIDS, effectively removing it from the electoral arena. Another possibility for a party to carry that political cost is to rely on an overwhelming electoral majority and steadfast loyalty of its voters. In the first case parties do not contest elections on the HIV/AIDS issue and in the second the government wins elections despite an initially unpopular policy on HIV/AIDS (for which it will be rewarded later). Consider figure 2 in this context.

Figure 2. HIV prevalence Thailand, Uganda, South Africa,1990-2000

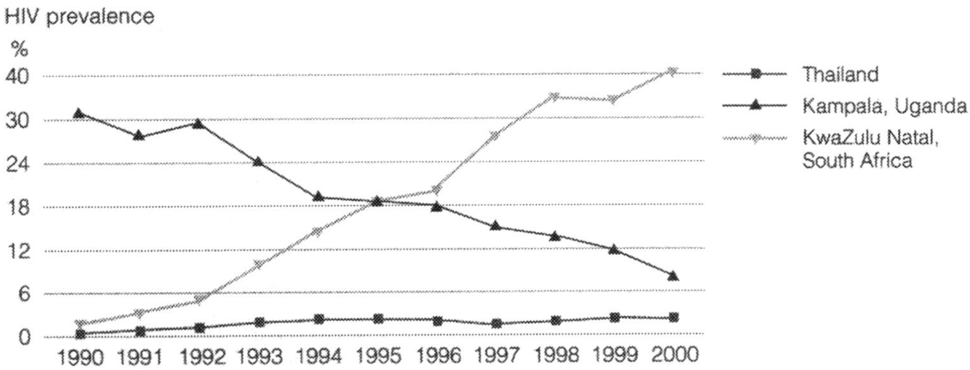

The graph shows the development of HIV prevalence rates in three different countries that represent three different political responses to the epidemic. The Thai government, which was non-democratic for parts of the relevant period, reacted strongly to early indications of the epidemic and has since managed to keep prevalence rates low. The Ugandan government, which still has to introduce competitive elections and many of the institutions of liberal democracy, reacted strongly to the shock that prevalence rates were very high and has since managed to reduce them considerably.

The two South African governments during the 1990s – the non-democratic apartheid government and the ANC government after the 1994 election – on the other hand responded relatively late to early signs of the epidemic and its policies have not yet had a marked effect on prevalence rates. These differences between the countries' responses need complex analyses where, for instance, culture, political transition and regime type all play into the explanation, but irrespective of these differences, the one similarity between the two successful cases is strong political leadership in combating the epidemic, something that has been interrogated in South Africa throughout the 1990s (Van Der Vliet, 2004). The context and contents of HIV/AIDS policies in South Africa will be explored further in chapter six. We shall round off this section by simply noting that for a variety of reasons political leaders in South Africa did not manage to formulate and launch a strong political response to the epidemic when there was still time to block the virus from causing an epidemic. They could not mobilise against the political incentives of the day; they were, indeed, busy birthing South Africa's democracy. Today, more than 10 years into the epidemic, it remains to be seen to what extent people's experiences of and attitudes towards the HIV/AIDS epidemic presents politicians with incentives in favour of a strong response against HIV/AIDS. In other words are there indications that suggest HIV/AIDS is now an issue with a direct impact on electoral outcomes; can it make or break a government?

2.2 TESTING SOUTH AFRICANS FOR HIV PREVALENCE

There are three authoritative sources of information on the national estimate of HIV infection in South Africa: the antenatal clinic data generated by the Department of Health (DoH, 2002), the survey data collected by the Human Sciences Research Council (HSRC) (Shisana 2002) and the estimates generated by the ASSA2000 model that builds in part on the antenatal clinic data (Dorrington 2002: Dorrington 2004). In our review and commentary below we shall refer to all three of these estimates wherever possible.

The most commonly cited estimate on HIV prevalence is generated through blood tests on a sample of the women who visit antenatal clinics provided by the public health care system, so called antenatal clinic tests. This method is used by the South African DoH and is relied on by a number of international organisations, most prominently UNAIDS. The DoH has conducted 14 annual tests since 1990. During October every year HIV tests are done on blood taken from a representative sample of all women who visit public clinics for the first time in their current pregnancy. The women are asked if they wish to participate in the HIV tests and it is very rare that women decline to give blood for this purpose. Once the blood is taken and the testing is done there is no way of tracing the sample back to the women who gave the blood. The strengths of this method is that the HIV test in itself is very reliable and that the "response rate" is close to 100%, meaning that all of the sampled women and clinics do indeed provide the necessary information to generate an estimate. Confidence intervals around the estimates are two percentages or less for women who are below 35 years and slightly more than two percentages, at the most 3.5 percentages, for women over 35 years. There are, however, three main disadvantages with this methodology. The first is a "fertility bias" since HIV-positive women are less fertile and therefore under-represented among the women who visit the clinics (Evian 2003).

For this reason the estimates might under-represent somewhat the true levels of HIV prevalence in the population. The second is that the women who visit the clinics are not a representative sample of all South African women. Around 80% of pregnant women visit these clinics, but these women are overwhelmingly from the relatively poorer black and coloured population groups, while a majority of Indian and white women visit private clinics. Another bias in the sample is that while the estimate is said to represent women 15-49 years old, less than 3% of the sampled women are over 40 years old, which makes the estimate for that age cohort less reliable. The assumptions that are applied to compensate for such an unrepresentative sample of women, and also to compensate for the complete lack of men in the sample, are in themselves a third disadvantage since they are more or less problematic and contestable, something that the DoH is careful to point out:

> *The Department of Health developed a model for estimating the number of HIV infected people in the general South African population based on the results of the survey. Certain assumptions are made and the results arrived at are only crude estimates due to the constraints of the survey. The estimates are only as good as the validity of the assumptions and the generalisability of the survey results, which are used in the extrapolation process (DoH, 2002: 4).*

The four critical assumptions made by the South African DoH are:

- The prevalence rate of HIV infection in all pregnant women in South Africa is the same as the prevalence rate in women attending public antenatal clinics;
- The prevalence rate of HIV infection in all women aged 15 to 49 years is the same as the prevalence rate in pregnant women;
- The estimate of infected males equals 85% of infected females;
- The mother-to-child transmission rate is 30% (DoH, 2002).

Needless to say, while the antenatal clinic method no doubt generates the most accurate estimate of HIV infection among pregnant women who visits public antenatal clinics, it is less reliable in estimating HIV prevalence for other groups of women and for the population as a whole. In our further references to these antenatal clinic estimates we therefore rely on them only to provide information about women in the actual "population", that is women who attend the clinics.

The second more direct method is the household survey where a nationally representative sample of households are visited and individuals are asked to answer a set of questions, as well as to do an HIV test. This method has become increasingly feasible with the development of a test for HIV that is based on a person's saliva, thus allowing a safe, fast and less intrusive means for testing than drawing blood. This household survey method was used for the first time in South Africa in 2001-2002 in a joint research project by the HSRC and the Nelson Mandela Foundation. The clear advantage of this method is that the sample is representative of the whole population. It thus generates estimates for a number of different segments of the population, as defined for instance by gender, age and race. The disadvantage with the method tends to be a low response rate, especially when people are asked and tested for something which is as filled with stigma as HIV and AIDS. The HSRC survey had a general response rate – that is, the percentage of people in the sample who agreed to be both interviewed and to leave a saliva specimen for HIV testing – of 62.3 percent (n = 13 518). This figure was, however, only around 55 percent for young and adult Indian South Africans (n = 647) and as low as 46.4% for white South Africans (n = 701). The effect of such low response rates is that the estimates for those population segments are relatively imprecise with wide confidence intervals, sometimes as wide as over 10 percentages (Shisana 2002). The South African household survey was also biased against those without a household at a permanent address, thus under-representing destitute South Africans among whom HIV prevalence tends to be higher.

The third method for generating a national HIV estimate, as well as much else relating to the epidemic, is a more theoretically complex and methodologically demanding statistical modelling. The most advanced of these models is the ASSA2000 model that has been developed by researchers at the Centre for Actuarial Research (CARE) at the University of Cape Town. The results from the DoH's antenatal clinic surveys since 1998 are factored into a complex statistical model that also takes a host of other demographic, developmental and health-related factors into account. These data are then processed on the basis of a set of epidemiological and demographic assumptions, all of which generate projections of for instance past, present and future levels of HIV prevalence, numbers of people sick with AIDS-related illnesses and mortality statistics due to AIDS. While this statistically sophisticated method can generate a wider range of estimates about the epidemic than the other two methods, its generated projections are of course only as reliable as the data fed into the model and to the extent that the assumptions that are made are reasonable. A problem with using the projections of the model in this regard is that the process by which they have been generated lacks transparency.

The main point we wish to make in conclusion is that in reviewing and relying on different estimates and projections of HIV prevalence one needs to be aware of their respective uncertainties, biases and assumptions while not allowing these to undermine the basic message that is put across by all methods of estimation: that the epidemic is rife and is ravaging the South African society (Bourne, 2003). The different sources of data are clear enough to motivate the strongest possible response to prevent further infections and to make HIV a chronic but manageable infection through effective treatment.

2.2.1 HOW DOES THE EPIDEMIC VARY IN THE POPULATION?

The most recent epidemiological update from the UNAIDS estimates that a total of 5.3 million South Africans are infected by the HI virus, a figure that surpasses those of all other countries (UNAIDS, 2004).[3] This figure translates to 11.4% of the total South African population of 46.6 million, a percentage that perfectly matches the estimate of national prevalence generated by the HSRC household survey (see table 1).

Table 1. Estimated national prevalence by age, race and gender. HSRC household survey 2002

Population Age segment	older than 2		15-24		15-49		25 and older	
Black	12.9	(11.2-14.5)	10.2	(7.9-12.5)	18.4	(15.5-20.5)	18.8	(16.2-21.3)
White	6.2	(3.1-9.2)	3.2	(0-7.5)	6.2	(4.0-11.5)	5.7	(2.7-8.7)
Coloured	6.1	(4.5-7.8)	6.4	(4.5-8.4)	6.6	(5.0-10.2)	6.7	(4.4-8.9)
Indian	1.6	(0-3.4)	0.3	(0.2-0.3)	1.8	(0.5-8.5)	2.3	(1.5-3.1)
Male	9.5	(8.0-11.1)	6.1	(3.9-8.3)	12.8	(10.5-15.2)	14.4	(11.6-17.1)
Female	12.8	(10.9-14.6)	12.0	(9.2-14.7)	17.7	(15.2-21.0)	16.2	(13.6-18..8)
Total	11.4	(10.0-12.7)	9.3	(7.3-11.2)	15.6	(14.0-17.5)	15.5	(13.5-17.5)

Source: Shisana 2002:46, 48 - 51. Confidence intervals in brackets.

A few features of the data are particularly noticeable. Starting with the racial groups, the virus is by far the most prevalent within the black population, with in some instances as much as almost three times the infection rate of the second worst hit group.

Despite these differences, it should be emphasised that the epidemic is indeed affecting all four groups, contrary to the prejudiced and often racist argument that the epidemic is only a problem for black South Africans. We should note further that the confidence intervals at times overlap between some of the groups, making it impossible to say with certainty that prevalence levels actually differ between those groups. A second observation is, as could be expected, that the prevalence rate is the highest in the age cohort that is most sexually active, that between 15 and 49 years of age. This age span is used internationally to define the "adult" population, the group the prevalence rates of which is most commonly cited. More importantly, a third observation is that women are considerably more affected than men, particularly in the younger age cohorts. It should be noted that the gender differences in the estimates are outside the margin of error in the two age cohorts that are most sexually active (15-24 and 15-49). A further breakdown of the statistics reveal even worse rates of infection for some women (see table 2).

Table 2. Prevalence among women (all/black) per age group

Age	15-19	20-24	25-29	30-34	35-39	40-44	45-49	Total
All women	7.3 (4.7-11.3)	17.1 (12.9-22.3)	32.0 (24.8-40.1)	24.1 (17.3-32.5)	13.8 (8.7-21.1)	19.0 (12.8-27.2)	11.2 (6.5-18.7)	17.7 (15.2-20.4)
Black women	7.5 (4.5-12.0)	19.1 (14.2-25.0)	38.6 (30.8-48.1)	29.7 (21.1-39.9)	17.5 (10.9-26.8)	22.5 (14.9-32.5)	11.3 (5.6-21.3)	20.7 (17.7-24.0)

Source: Shisana 2002:53. Confidence intervals in brackets.

When African (black) women between 15 and 49 years of age are singled out the average prevalence rate rises by three percentages to almost 21%. Note that black women here are compared with "all" women, a category that of course also includes black women. If black women instead were compared with women in the three other racial groups, the differences would become much starker. Such comparisons should, however, not be necessary to alert us to the alarming information that almost four out of every ten African women in their late twenties are HIV-positive. The important message here is that women are considerably more affected than men. This can be explained by both socio-political as well as by biological factors.

The woman is more vulnerable to infection during intercourse as her genital membranes are more easily penetrated by the virus than those of the man (Evian, 2003). Adding to this vulnerability is the fact that women, for cultural, social and political reasons, often are dominated by the man, making it impossible for them to negotiate safe sex (Baylies & Bujra, 1997; Campbell, 2003).

A natural point of comparison between the three estimates is to look at women of child-bearing age (15-49 years). The HSRC survey estimates HIV prevalence for this group to be 17.7%, which is the lowest of the three. Both the ASSA2000 model and the antenatal clinic data estimate it to be considerably higher at 25.9% and 27.9% respectively. A detailed breakdown of the estimates for antenatal clinic attendees (women 15-49 years of age) shows that the estimates based on the antenatal clinic data are higher for all age cohorts (see table 3).[4] The estimates by the DoH would most probably surpass the HSRC estimates also for 25-29 year old black women if the antenatal clinic data could distinguish between racial groups. Having said that, it also should be noted that the differences in estimates between the HSRC and the DoH are outside the margin of error only for the two youngest and the total group of women.

Table 3. Prevalence among ANC attendees in 2003, by age group

younger than 20	20-24	25-29	30-34	35-39	40+	Total
15.8 (28.8-31.8)	30.3 (33.6-37.2)	35.4 (28.9-32.9)	30.9 (20.9-25.9)	23.4 15.8	5.8 (12.3-19.3)	27.9 (26.8-28.9)

Source: DoH 2002:8. Confidence intervals in brackets.

In this section we have detailed differences between estimates of HIV prevalence, but also differences between population groups based on race and gender within the HSRC estimate. Before we continue it is important to note that while these percentages are the best available estimates of the extent of the epidemic, they do not at all reflect the level of awareness about one's HIV status in the population. On the contrary, according to the HSRC survey, as many as 76% of HIV-positive South Africans are not aware of being infected (Shisana, 2002).

To increase this awareness – to make sure everyone knows his/her HIV status – would not only mean that the lives of those who are infected might be prolonged through medication as well as save the health and lives of those who risk being infected by them, but it would also generate a constituency that potentially could do much constructive advocacy in communities and in relation to political institutions to break down stigma and apply pressure for a strong and effective political response; a point to which we will return in later chapters.

2.2.2 WHERE ARE RATES OF INFECTION THE HIGHEST?

Another relevant aspect of the epidemic for our inquiry relates to variations in estimated prevalence between the nine provinces. Our three sources of epidemiological data differ a great deal in the estimates they present for levels of HIV prevalence in the nine provinces (see table 4). The estimates by ASSA2000 and the DoH are the most similar as they build on the same antenatal clinic data, but the estimates generated in the household survey are in some instances radically different. KwaZulu-Natal stands out in particular, with an estimate from DoH that is more than twice as high as that from the HSRC.

Table 4. Population and three estimates of HIV prevalence, by provinces

Province	SA population mid-2004, %		Prevalence 2002 in % by ASSA2000 *	Prevalence 2003 in % by DoH **		Prevalence 2002 in % by HSRC ***	
Western Cape	4 570 696	9.8	6.7	13.1	(8.5-17.7)	13.2	(8.0-20.0)
Eastern Cape	7 088 547	15.2	20.5	27.1	(24.6-29.7)	10.2	(7.0-14.0)
Northern Cape	899 349	1.9	12.9	16.7	(11.9-21.5)	9.6	(6.5-14.5)
Free State	2 950 661	6.3	26.5	30.1	(26.9-33.3)	19.4	(14.0-27.5)
KwaZulu-Natal	9 665 875	20.7	31.4	37.5	(35.2-39.8)	15.7	(12.0-21.5)
North West	3 807 469	8.2	24.8	29.9	(26.8-33.1)	14.4	(10.0-19.5)
Gauteng	8 847 740	19.0	23.8	29.6	(27.8-31.5)	20.3	(16.0-25.3)
Mpumalanga	3 244 306	7.0	28.1	32.6	(28.5-36.6)	21.0	(15.0-28.0)
Limpopo	5 511 962	11.9	20.9	17.5	(14.9-20.0)	11.5	(7.5-17.0)
National	**46 586 607**	**100.1**	**23.4**	**27.9**	**(26.8-28.9)**	11.4	(10.1-12.7)

Sources: Statistics SA 2004: 31-32; Dorrington 2002: 5; Shisana 2002: 50; DoH 2002:7. Confidence intervals in brackets.

* Prevalence among ages 18-64 years; ** Prevalence among ANC attendees, 15-49 years; *** Prevalence among ages 15-49 years.

Since our research will seek to establish whether there are any general patterns of correlations, we can allow some simplification of this data and look at how the nine provinces can be ranked according to their levels of HIV prevalence. In addition to such a simplification of the differences between the estimates generated by the three methodologies, we shall also note which of the differences in estimates by the DoH and the HSRC are outside the margin of error.

Table 5. Ranking of provinces by estimated HIV prevalence

Province	ASSA2000	DoH	HSRC	Outside the margin of error
Western Cape	9	9	6	No
Eastern Cape	7	6	8	Yes
Northern Cape	8	8	9	No
Free State	3	3	3	No
KwaZulu-Natal	1	1	4	Yes
North West	4	4	5	Yes
Gauteng	5	5	2	Yes
Mpumalanga	2	2	1	Yes
Limpopo	6	7	7	No

Sources: See table 4 above. 1 indicates the highest estimate and 9 indicates the lowest estimate.

When we look beyond the detail of estimated percentages of prevalence, we start instead to see similarities between the different estimates; two provinces are ranked similarly by the DoH and the HSRC; the same four provinces are ranked among the four with the lowest estimates; and the differences are within the margin of error in four cases. While this simplification of the data hides important nuances in it, the purpose here has been to show that the differences between the provinces are reduced when we look at the more general picture.

2.2.3 AIDS-RELATED SICKNESS AND DEATHS

When we discuss and perhaps make demands on certain policies from a democratic government to combat HIV/AIDS we need to remember that our most basic and principled expectation of democracy as a political system cannot be that it has particular foresight about future problems or that it is especially effective in dealing with them, but that it is responsive to citizens' demands as their needs change over time. One could argue that while foresight and effectiveness are favourable characteristics of any form of government, responsiveness is a necessary quality for a democracy to be sustainable over time. The implication of this reasoning for our discussion here is that a democratic government at the very least needs to be responsive and react to the frustration and devastation in society caused by increasing numbers of people falling ill and dying from AIDS-related diseases. If it fails to respond to such demands it is less democratic than it could be and risks being undermined by the very problem it refuses to address.

An inquiry into AIDS-related sickness and death quickly runs into problems with data. Statistics SA keeps records of mortality in South Africa and the latest released data record deaths up until the year 2000, but there is no way of distinguishing whether AIDS was the cause of death (Statistics SA, 2001). Statistics SA notes further that its data will under-represent the total number of deaths since some, and particularly so in the poorer and more marginalised communities where AIDS is more prevalent, are never reported to the authorities. Consider table 6.

Table 6. Recorded deaths by province, 1997-2000

Province	1997	%	1998	%	1999	%	2000	%
Western Cape	29 384	11.4	31 585	10.7	32 787	10.2	34 390	9.7
Eastern Cape *	30 248	11.7	36 947	12.5	43 615	13.6	49 832	14.0
Northern Cape	7 792	3.0	8 364	2.8	8 749	2.7	9†414	2.6
Free State	23 055	8.9	26 493	9.0	28 842	9.0	31 423	8.8
KwaZulu-Natal *	57 533	22.3	67 313	22.8	75 206	23.4	84 851	23.8
North West *	18 286	7.1	21 330	7.2	25 036	7.8	28 940	8.1
Gauteng	55 564	21.6	61 040	20.6	62 506	19.4	67 587	19.0
Mpumalanga	17 738	6.9	20 344	6.9	22 577	7.0	25 002	7.0
Northern Province	18 227	7.1	22 415	7.6	22 192	6.9	24 775	7.0
Total	**257 827**	**100**	**295 831**	**100**	**321 510**	**100**	**356 214**	**100**

Source: Statistics SA 2001: 3. * Provinces with a clear trend of an increasing share of deaths nationally.

The ASSA2000 model provides us with more relevant data with its projections of the numbers of AIDS sick and AIDS-related deaths by province (see table 7).

Table 7. Projected AIDS sick and AIDS deaths, by province

Province	AIDS sick in 2004, % of total population *	Projected total AIDS deaths 1990-2004, % of total population *
Western Cape	0.38	0.64
Eastern Cape	1.10	1.90
Northern Cape	0.73	1.17
Free State	2.74	3.38
KwaZulu-Natal	2.31	4.56
North West	1.62	2.90
Gauteng	1.78	3.13
Mpumalanga	2.05	4.17
Limpopo	1.10	1.98
National	**1.57**	**2.90**

Source: Dorrington 2002: 10-28.* Total population refers to the projected total provincial population in the ASSA2000 model.

The term "AIDS sick" implies that a person has entered stage four of the disease, with a CD4 count of less than 200, when s/he is so severely affected by AIDS-related illnesses that s/he is bedridden for considerable periods of time. Arguably, two possible explanations for the differences between the provinces in this regard are the length of time during which the epidemic has been affecting the provincial population and the general state of health of that population; the "older" the epidemic is, the higher the number of AIDS sick will be, and the healthier the provincial population, the lower the number of AIDS sick will be. The same general logic presumably applies in explaining the differences in how many people have died from AIDS-related illnesses in proportion to the provincial population. Data on poverty – as a proxy for "provincial health" – seem to corroborate this interpretation. Both the HDI and the HPI (poverty indicators that will be introduced in the next section) correlate accordingly with the variations in AIDS-related sickness and death in the different provinces.[5] The relevance of these projections for our research will become clearer further below and in chapter seven as we test two hypotheses on the impact of the epidemic on public opinion and the electoral processes.

2.2.4 POVERTY AND THE EPIDEMIC

The obvious next step in the analysis after having identified how the epidemic varies over population segments and provinces would be to seek explanations to those variations. However, to do this in a systematic way – even in terms of a literary review – would lead us too far off our course in the present inquiry. To the extent that we have an explanatory ambition in our research the causal arrow points to the opposite direction; we will test whether the epidemic can explain variations in the data on voter registration and voter turnout in the 2004 elections. The results from these tests will be presented and discussed in chapter eight, but they need to be prefaced here by a discussion of the one other structural variable that might prove to be relevant as a competing or complementary explanation – levels of poverty.

Poverty is particularly relevant for our inquiry since it has been identified in the social science literature on the epidemic as one of a few crucial structural variables with a direct impact on various facets of the epidemic (Fredland, 1998; Whiteside, 2002). The Human Development Index (HDI) is an instrument for measuring the wellbeing of people by combining indices on life expectancy, educational attainment and gross domestic product. It can vary between 0 and 1, where values between 1 and .8 are interpreted as high human development, values between .799 and .5 are medium level and values below .499 indicate low levels of human development. For a number of years the United Nations Development Programme (UNDP) has produced reports in which it ranks the countries of the world according to their respective HDI scores. When we compare the scores from 1996 and 2003 for a number of Southern African countries, all of which are severely affected by the epidemic, we can see that all countries have fallen on that ranking (see table 8). One obvious explanation for this is the detrimental effect the epidemic has on life expectancy, which in some instances dropped some 20 years between 1996 and 2003. The further counterfactual experiment to project life expectancy with and without the impact of AIDS shows the detrimental impact of the epidemic with even more brutal clarity. For instance, if prevention does not succeed and treatment does not effectively halt the lethal effect of the virus, Botswana is projected to see its life expectancy reduced from 70 to 29 years by the year 2010, effectively wiping out decades of development that has elevated Botswana to one of the strongest economies and most consolidated democracies on the continent. It is important to note that this discussion and the projections in the literature that are presented in the table below are not true statements of reality, but counterfactual statements of what life expectancy would be if, on the one hand, there was no AIDS in the population and, on the other hand, what life expectancy will be if no efforts were made to stop the effect of AIDS. The point is that both theses statements are untrue; AIDS causes deaths but since governments and societies have responded to the challenge, the non-intervention scenarios are no longer relevant. The scenarios are, arguably, nevertheless still relevant as stark reminders of the threat posed by the epidemic.

Table 8. AIDS-related statistics and projections from selected countries in Southern Africa

	UNDP 1996 A		UNDP 2003 A		LE 2000 B		LE 2010 B		Adult prevalence C
	LE	HDI	LE	HDI	AIDS	No AIDS	AIDS	No AIDS	
Botswana	65.0	71	44.7	125	39.3	70.5	29	70.3	37.3
Malawi	45.5	157	38.5	162	37.6	53.3	35.8	57.3	14.2
Namibia	59.1	116	47.4	124	-	-	-	-	22.3
South Africa	63.2	100	50.9	111	51.1	65.7	35.5	68.3	21.5
Swaziland	57.8	110	38.2	133	-	-	-	-	38.8
Zambia	48..6	136	33.4	163	37.2	58.9	38.9	62.8	16.5
Zimbabwe	53.4	124	35.4	145	37.8	69.9	32.2	72.8	24.6

Source: A Whiteside & Barnett, 2002, citing UNDP and the US Bureau of the Census, B UNDP, 2003. C Estimates for end of 2003, UNAIDS, 2004.

A more comprehensive and detailed account of current levels of poverty in South Africa is provided by the UNDP in its *South Africa Human Development Report 2003*. With the subtitle *The Challenge of Sustainable Development in South Africa: Unlocking People's Creativity* the UNDP captures the dilemma that poverty presents to South Africa. Despite a decade of successfully sustaining and consolidating its democratic regime, the country has yet to find ways of "unlocking" the full creative potential of those of its citizens who are still trapped in poverty. Unless this unused pool of human resources is channelled and developed creatively, the social foundations for the democratic regime as such will increasingly be undermined. The problem that the UNDP clarifies is that many of the crucial indicators are pointing to negative trends. People's potential is not being "unlocked". On the contrary, more people find themselves increasingly locked into the traps of poverty, see table 9.

Table 9. Poverty indicators for South Africa, by gender, race and province

		Poverty % A		Poverty B gap %		Gini C		HDI D		HPI E	
		1995	2002	1995	2002	1995	2001	1995	2003	1995	2001
	National	51.1	48.5	17.8	18.0	.595	.635	.740	.660	16.0	22.0
Gender	Female	53.4	50.9	18.4	18.2	.560	.600	–	–	15.5	21.5
	Male	48.9	45.9	17.1	17.8	.580	..625	–	–	17.5	22.5
Race	Black	62.0	56.3	22.1	21.5	..540	.575	–	–	19.0	25.5
	White	1.5	6.9	1.5	2.4	..465	475	–	–	3.5	4.5
	Coloured	38.5	36.1	10.7	11.6	.490	.555	–	–	9.5	12.0
	Indian	8.3	14.7	2.2	4..4	.440	.520	–	–	5.0	5.5
Provinces	Western Cape	28.6	28.8	7.5	8.5	.540	.590	.790	.760	9.5	12.0
	Eastern Cape	71.2	68.3	26.9	27.9	.610	.655	.670	.620	23.0	24.0
	Northern Cape	55.4	54.4	19.0	19.6	.600	.630	.720	.690	16.5	17.0
	Free State	63.6	59.9	20.9	20.3	.625	.645	.745	.670	14.5	22..5
	KwaZulu-Natal	53.2	50.5	18.1	18.9	.565	.610	.710	.625	16.5	27.0
	North West	59.4	56.5	22.4	21.9	.595	.585	.675	.605	23.0	25.0
	Gauteng	18.4	20.0	6.2	7.9	.530	.615	.810	.740	10..5	19.0
	Mpumalanga	59.7	54.8	20.9	20.0	.560	.610	.725	.650	19.5	26.0
	Limpopo	62.7	60.7	23.7	23.5	.640	..600	.640	.595	20.5	22.0

A) Income poverty: percent of adults who live on less than R354 per month. B) Income poverty gap: the mean shortfall of R354, in percent of that sum. C) Gini-coefficient: measures the extent of income inequality where 0 is perfect equality and 1 is perfect inequality. D) Human Development Index: a composite index of indices of life expectancy, educational attainment and gross domestic product, where 0 is low development and 1 is high development. E) Human Poverty Index: a combined index of three indicators of poverty: the probability at birth of not surviving to age 40, adult literacy rate, and the percentages of people not using improved water sources and children under five who are underweight where higher numbers indicate higher levels of poverty.
Source: UNDP 2003: 41-46.

The first measurement, income poverty has decreased somewhat overall except for relatively large increases in the white and Indian population groups and in the Gauteng province. The national decrease of 2.6 percentages is, however, less than the growth of the population; there were more people living in poverty in 2002 than in 1995. The "poverty gap" presents a mixed picture. Some of those living under the poverty line have become a little less poor, whereas others are dropping further below that line. The strongest improvement was seen in Mpumalanga (by .9 percentages) and the largest drops can be found in Gauteng and in the Indian population (1.7 and 2.2 percentages respectively). The last three indicators are more complex in their construction with more obvious political implications as they reveal the stark inequalities in the South African society and show more directly the extent to which people struggle with poverty and underdevelopment. Of all the different categories brought out by UNDP, the level of inequality has increased in all but two provinces (North West and Limpopo). South Africa is an increasingly unequal society. The levels of human development are decreasing in all the provinces (data were not provided for the other categories) and, perhaps most problematically, levels of human poverty are increasing in all categories. It is worth reflecting a bit more on the realities that are represented by this last indicator. What it tells us is that, in 2001, seven years into South Africa's hard-won democracy, people are, on balance, struck more by poverty than they were a year after the transition. The complexities of explaining this observation are of course enormous. Some would even challenge the validity of the UNDP's indicator. Taking these complexities and arguments into account, we do not intend these comments to challenge any particular claims by the South African government of having improved the living conditions for South Africans (South African Government 2003). What we are saying, however, is that to the extent that poverty fuels the HIV/AIDS epidemic, the macro indicators of poverty are suggesting that this structural context to the epidemic is increasingly undermining any other government interventions to deal constructively with the epidemic.

But what support is there in our data for the argument that poverty fuels the epidemic? If the general hypothesis is correct and if it applies to the South African context we would expect positive correlations between the levels of HIV prevalence and levels of poverty. Is it, given the data we have available to us, the case that provinces with higher levels of poverty also have higher levels of HIV prevalence and AIDS sickness? Correlation analyses of the different variables yield results that give some statistical support for the argument. There is no correlation between the more direct income poverty indicators or the Gini-coefficient and HIV prevalence; those instruments are too blunt. It is only with the indicators that are based on more substantial representations of poverty that we find a pattern. The HIV estimates from the HSRC did not, however, respond even to these indicators, but there was considerable correlation with the other two estimates. The correlation (Pearson's r) between the DoH estimates and the HDI is -.364, and a high .827 with the HPI. The correlations between the ASSA2000 estimates and these to poverty indicators are extraordinarily high (.55 and .91 respectively).[6]

Our analysis has clearly demonstrated the relevance of including poverty as a contextual variable in any social science discussion on the epidemic (Whiteside 2002). We can logically see why poverty fuels the epidemic, but we have also made the link statistically by establishing a correlation between HIV prevalence and levels of human development and human poverty among the nine provinces in South Africa.

CONCLUSION

Our review of some relevant information on the epidemic in South Africa generates a few general conclusions. The most obvious comment is that, irrespective of whether we rely on antenatal clinic data or survey data or data generated by a statistical model, the epidemic is very serious indeed. Two of the epidemic's three "waves" are now seriously affecting the South African society: HIV prevalence is still extremely high among large parts of the population and those who contracted the virus a number of years ago are now dying in increasing numbers. According to Alan Whiteside's theory of the epidemiological waves, we should now also start seeing how its third wave has an increasing impact on the economy and society more generally. We now turn to investigating how this impact in the third wave of the epidemic can impact on electoral processes more generally and whether an impact from the epidemic could be discerned in the April 2004 elections in South Africa.

It is very important… to note how the UNDP regards the relation between the two concepts 'governance' and 'democratic governance.' While one can identify good and bad governance, democratic governance is not a sub-set of good governance. The UNDP is very clear in saying that '[from] a human development perspective, good governance is democratic governance' (UNDP 2002cb: 51). Clearly then there are only two kinds of governance – there is bad governance and there is democratic governance.

CHAPTER 3

HIV/AIDS AND DEMOCRATIC GOVERNANCE

3.1 INTRODUCTION

One of the many cherished qualities that distinguish a democracy from other political regimes is that those in power have to be sensitive and responsive to the needs of the people to remain in power. The concerns, aspirations and fears that are held by citizens can find expression in an environment of open and critical public debate and find representation through civil society activism or political party policy. The power of such demands can be determined either by the moral principles that are at stake or by the numbers of people who back them up, or both. When faced with such demands, a democracy will react, policy will change and an administration will start working according to its new political directives. Political leaders thus make themselves accountable for well-balanced and effective political interventions that are responsive to popular demand while also taking other constitutional, political, financial and practical considerations into account. Politicians are rewarded or sanctioned as the electorate expresses its judgements of those interventions in free and fair elections. This is the case in theory; this is the ideal of democratic governance.

The magnitude of the HIV/AIDS pandemic in southern Africa represents an enormous challenge to the societies and democracies in the region. The complexity of the problem ranges from how the virus constantly mutates to avoid its antidote, to the structural violence of poverty that makes individuals more prone to infection and so vulnerable that treatment might cause as much harm as the virus. With prevalence levels in some places exceeding 30%, any democratic government, any economy and any society would take serious strain in trying to respond to this threat. Where resources are relatively limited and neither government nor civil society has had much time to practise democracy or become steeped in its culture of tolerance and accountability, this challenge might prove too difficult and threaten democracy itself (Hope, 1999; Willan, 2000). The main purpose of the discussion in this chapter is to show what the links are between the epidemic and the ideals and practices of democratic governance. What does democratic governance mean in general and what in particular does it imply in the context of the epidemic? How is the epidemic a threat to democratic governance? And how does the democratic electoral process fit in to this discussion?

3.2 DEFINITIONS AND DIMENSIONS OF DEMOCRATIC GOVERNANCE

As with most complex concepts in the public discourse, "democratic governance" holds many and sometimes confusing definitions. We therefore need to unpack the notion of democratic governance and see what its various more theoretical and practical dimensions are to understand properly its application in the discussion on HIV/AIDS and the South African election.

3.2.1 GOVERNANCE IN THEORY

The concept of governance has arguably some advantages over related concepts.[7] Different from "government", it does not focus our attention solely on the political elites with power to run the state, be they elected or not, but issues of governance are also relevant within civil society. And whereas "policy-making" captures the political process of formulating the substance of government intervention, governance also relates to the institutional arrangements that structure that political process. To shed further clarity Göran Hyden (1992) identifies four dimensions of the concept. Firstly, governance assumes that political dynamics have a basis in human agency; that politics is the result of the action and interaction of individuals in pursuit of ideals and interests. But, unlike competing paradigms, it does not assume that these individuals are competing in a zero-sum game where one's gain is another's loss. Instead governance recognises the potential of politics as "a positive-sum game; where reciprocal behaviour and legitimate relations of power between governors and governed prevail; and where everybody is a winner not only in the short term but also in the long run" ((Hyden 1992: 10). In other words governance assumes the possibility of formulating political solutions that are stable over time, not because of the domination of one interest over the other but because parties have found common ground through a co-operative process.

Secondly, governance seeks out a middle way between a structural approach that emphasises how political actors are governed by circumstances outside their control, and the rational approach which assumes that actors can negotiate and change any such circumstances to better suit their needs. The important research agenda which is suggested by governance is rather to understand how these two approaches complement each other in shaping politics. The third dimension is a governance realm that is defined by the first two dimensions: governance assumes that legitimate authority is respected since it is applied carefully to maintain reciprocal exchanges among people and incentives are conducive to entrenching trust between people since power is held accountable.

When it is conceptualised in this manner, governance generates good politics per definition. But Hyden *et al* also elaborate on a fourth dimension of the concept: a normatively neutral and empirical investigation of the quality of governance in different political regimes. In this perspective, when governance is

> *defined as regime management, governance is concerned with how rules (or structures) affect political action and the prospects of solving given societal problems. For much of the time, governance means the mere sustenance of the regime, but the real test of governance comes in situations where regime changes are needed to meet new demands or deal with new problems. ... The study of governance, then, involves the identification of the conditions that facilitate good governance and, by implication, effective problem solving (Hyden 1992:14-15).*

Hyden proposes three criteria for what constitutes good governance: the degree to which citizens can have influence on and oversight of the political process; the degree to which leadership is responsive and responsible; and the degree to which interactions in civil society are characterised by social reciprocities, ie equality, tolerance and inclusiveness. The point here is that the concept of governance does carry a normative bias in the more theoretical academic discourse; political power generates good results when it is applied according to governance principles. But it is left to empirical investigation to explore whether an actual regime is governed in such a way; the concept can be operationalised into a set of criteria that help us determine the degree to which a regime complies with governance ideals.

In empirical inquiries into how regimes respond to HIV/AIDS it would thus seem particularly relevant and potentially very fruitful to apply the concept of governance. The epidemic puts regimes to the test like few other challenges. It is of a magnitude that denies regimes the comfort of relying on normal procedures and will demand a reprioritisation of resources; in brief it requires nothing less than good governance.

3.2.2 GOVERNANCE AND DEVELOPMENT

The concept of governance gained prominence in the literature by featuring in a 1989 World Bank report that identified poor governance to be the problem with development in Africa. Corruption, nepotism and personalisation of power – or neo-patrimonial rule – were all practices that undermined any hopes for long-term sustainable development. The argument was that unless African countries became democratic there was little hope for the continent. Up to 15 years later we now know that, on the whole, a quick shot of liberal democratic institutions has made little difference in terms of alleviating poverty and generating development, but this has not reduced the prominence of the governance concept in the literature. Subsequent to the World Bank report, it is primarily the United Nations Development Programme (UNDP) that has developed and applied the concept further. In a UNDP report from 1997, *Reconceptualising Governance*, the UNDP elaborates on four different types of governance: economic, political, administrative and systemic. Political governance, being most relevant to our discussion here,[8] "refers to decision-making and policy implementation of a legitimate and authoritative state. The state should consist of separate legislative, executive and judicial branches, represent the interests of a pluralist polity, and allow citizens to freely elect their representatives" (UNDP 1997:10). Clearly this set of institutions and procedures is not only "political" but also "democratic", but at this stage the UNDP maintains the more generic term. And further, this qualitative requirement of governance is merely postulated as having positive effects on human development, no empirical analysis is provided to back up the argument.

It is not until its 2002 Human Development Report, *Deepening Democracy in a Fragmented World*, that the UNDP identifies *democratic* governance and discusses why the democratic aspect is necessary for human development on the basis of empirical evidence (UNDP 2002a). In a separate research paper for the main report the authors elaborate:

> *Like the concept of "good governance", democratic governance seeks efficient institutions, and a predictable economic and political environment necessary for economic growth and effective functioning of public services. But the concept of democratic governance shares with humane governance the concerns with political freedom and human rights, and removal of discrimination as central objectives. A reform agenda would aim not only at building institutions and rules that are not just efficient but also fair, and that are developed through a democratic process in which all people have a real political voice. Democratic governance thus incorporates into the notion of good governance for development, democratic processes, and a concern with the securing of political and civil rights and freedoms as human rights. Democratic governance differs from the concept of "good governance" in recognizing that political and civil freedoms and participation have intrinsic value as developmental ends in themselves. They are not just means for achieving socio-economic progress (Fukuda-Parr & Ponzio 2002: 5-6).*

It is clear that the introduction of "democratic governance" into this development discourse infuses central principles of political liberalism – protecting individuals' rights against the political ambitions of the developmental state – into a discourse that for some time has been dominated by other ideological paradigms. However, and somewhat contradictory, the UNDP's understanding of the concept departs from the liberal paradigm in that it prescribes substantive outcomes for the political process and a large role for the state in seeking to realise an ideal society on behalf of the citizens. This is clear from the check list that the authors provide on what democratic governance means:

- People's human rights and fundamental freedoms are respected, allowing them to live with dignity;
- People have a say in decisions that affect their lives;
- People can hold decision-makers accountable;
- Inclusive and fair rules, institutions and practices govern social interactions;
- Women are equal partners with men in private and public spheres of life and decision-making;
- People are free from discrimination based on race, ethnicity, class, gender or any other attribute;
- The needs of future generations are reflected in current policies;
- Economic and social policies are responsive to people's needs and aspirations;
- Economic and social policies aim at eradicating poverty and expanding the choices that all people have in their lives. (Fukuda-Parr & Ponzio, 2002: 6)

A list like this can be interpreted in at least two ways. In one reading the list sets out a number of thresholds that a polity has to pass before its political practice and processes can be characterised as democratic governance. If so, the stated criteria are minimum values on the different "variables" that comprise democratic governance. The alternative reading is that they rather represent maximum values, ie that they are statements of ideals that hardly, if ever, can be achieved. If so, democratic governance is an ideal that real polities can only approximate. The authors – no doubt very authoritative people in their field – are not quite clear on which interpretation they intend. If anything their writing suggests it is a list of thresholds. But on a practical level the problem remains the same, irrespective of which interpretation we apply: democratic governance is unrealistic either because it is too difficult to achieve (which democracy fulfils such criteria?) or because the criteria intentionally were placed beyond reach.

> *It is very important, finally, to note how the UNDP regards the relation between the two concepts "governance" and "democratic governance." While one can identify good and bad governance, democratic governance is not a sub-set of good governance. The UNDP is very clear in saying that "[from] a human development perspective, good governance is democratic governance" ((UNDP 2002cb: 51). Clearly then, there are only two kinds of governance – there is bad governance and there is democratic governance.*

There are two implications of this for our discussion here. Initially, and arguably, if these discussions are to have any practical implications, both the concept of democratic governance and any effort to list its constituent parts should be regarded as normative ideals, as certain political goals to strive for. In saying that, it is important to emphasise that they are normative and that they capture certain political goals. This is not to say that anyone would not want to see a world thoroughly transformed by a total and complete process of human development; a world where the UNDP's mission has been achieved. The contention rather lies in the prescribed ways of getting there. On the basis of the African experience, for instance, one could make the argument that human development is unlikely ever to be realised through democratic governance, if this necessarily implies a major role for the bureaucracies that make up the African states (Van de Walle, 2001). And to make matters worse, we shall see in section 3.2.3 below how the HIV/AIDS epidemic is most likely to further undermine efforts to introduce democratic governance in the African polities. Secondly, given that the agency defines good governance as democratic governance we would of course expect this to be reflected in its proposals for a governance response to the HIV/AIDS epidemic.

3.2.3 Governance responses to HIV/AIDS

Let us initially take stock of what our conceptual discussions above imply for our focus on governance and HIV/AIDS. The more theoretical discussions by Göran Hyden suggested that we must distinguish between a normative and an empirical investigation into governance. While the concept of governance is loaded with positive connotations, our empirical investigation into governance is based on an objective analytical framework that allows us to characterise to what degree a polity approximates the ideal. Such an analysis can be done when the polity is under no particular stress, but the analysis is all the more relevant when, as in the case of HIV/AIDS, the political system and civil society both have to find ways of dealing with a national crisis. The more practically oriented development discourse, ironically, proved to be less clear in how one should apply its definitions and arguments on democratic governance to existing political systems. Our interpretation is, in the end, that democratic governance should be the ideal for the whole of the political process across different development-related policy arenas, also in national crises like the HIV/AIDS epidemic.

If we for the moment stay with the argument that democratic governance is the only acceptable form of governance, what policy directives for fighting HIV/AIDS have been generated on that basis? We can list (from A to I) a number of governance related interventions and capacities that are suggested and emphasised by the UNDP (2002b). The organisation identifies three interrelated concepts as the basis for governance when dealing with HIV/AIDS: mainstreaming; a multi-sectoral response; and effective implementation. (A) *Mainstreaming* is understood as the response of a sector or department to two sets of questions: (1) What is the impact of HIV/AIDS on the organisation and its capacity to deliver on its mandate? What policies, strategies and actions have been, or could be, designed and implemented to minimise this impact?

(2) How does the organisation, in seeking to fulfil its mandate, affect the nature, manifestation and spread of the HIV/AIDS epidemic? What policies, strategies and actions have been, or could be, designed and implemented to minimise negative impacts and maximise positive impacts? Once these questions have been addressed by all parts of the administration, their responses need to be integrated into a (B) *multi-sectoral response* to HIV/AIDS with the intention of preventing further HIV transmission through behavioural change, providing care and treatment of people living with HIV/AIDS and mitigating current and future social and economic impacts of the epidemic. The third element is that (C) the *effective implementation* of a multi-sectoral response is contingent on a number of inter-dependent and mutually reinforcing conditions; (D) The *recognition* of HIV/AIDS as a development issue that necessitates a multi-sectoral response to HIV/AIDS; (E) Sufficient *institutional capacity* to conduct and analyse research, to develop and implement sectoral plans and to articulate and review appropriate interventions; (F) *Coordination* through the establishment of an appropriate organisational framework; (G) *Financial resources* to implement sectoral plans and relevant interventions; (H) *Stakeholder involvement* in the various stages of design, implementation, monitoring and evaluation of interventions; and (I) a *Monitoring and evaluation framework*, with clear and measurable indicators. In brief, a good governance response to HIV/AIDS is one that is permeated by an awareness of the epidemic and practical responses implemented successfully across all sectors of society. However, given our discussion above, the question is how we should understand this list of interventions. Are these also ideals, or more practical and realistic suggestions?

It is quite clear that the UNDP list that defines a governance response to the epidemic is a set of practical and quite realistic suggestions that can serve as a check list when an organisation or government needs to improve on its response to HIV/AIDS. The list does not contain idealistic formulations about certain political outcomes. While this approach, arguably, should be promoted, it unfortunately falls short of the more practical aspects of democratic governance; human rights and checks on power.

A comparison of the two lists above, between the one that defines democratic governance and the one that defines governance in response to HIV/AIDS, clearly exemplifies in what ways *democratic* governance adds critical dimensions and principles to the original term governance. The two points of vague correspondence are that both lists emphasise the need for people (or stakeholders) to be involved in governance processes and, by implication, that those who formulate governance interventions on HIV/AIDS must be held accountable in relation to an evaluation framework. However, even these two vague similarities could be challenged. To say, as in democratic governance, that *people should have a say in decisions that affect them* and that *people should be able to hold decision-makers accountable* are two central democratic commitments, whereas, as in governance on HIV/AIDS, to allow "stakeholders" some influence and to "evaluate" governance interventions' need not have much, if any, democratic content. It is unclear to these authors what we are to make of this important discrepancy between the UNDP's promotion of democratic governance more generally and their definition of a governance response to HIV/AIDS more specifically. There is of course no basis for believing that the UNDP would argue against a democratic governance response to HIV/AIDS since, given the definitions used by the UNDP, this would be tantamount to saying that bad governance should be the response to HIV/AIDS. We need more clarity from the UNDP.

The recent joint publication by UNAIDS and UNDP – *Building Dynamic Democratic Governance and HIV/Resilient Societies* – by Lee-Nah Hsu (2004), manager of the UNDP's HIV and Development Programme in South East Asia, seeks to provide additional clarity. Although the report is not an official policy statement, it is clearly an authoritative statement from a senior UNDP official which is bound to have an impact on the development of the discourse on democratic governance in relation to HIV/AIDS. The next section is a review of and comment on this document.

3.2.4 DEMOCRATIC GOVERNANCE RESPONSES TO HIV/AIDS

Democratic governance in relation to HIV/AIDS should, argues Hsu, build on three pillars (2004:3-4). Firstly, governance should be based on "*participation, responsiveness to all stakeholders and consensus orientation*". While there should be "mediation between differing interests to reach a broad consensus on the best interest of a group", such mediation must not be abused by non-committal politicians; democracy provides people with the power to "remove those who no longer reflect people's aspirations and concerns". Secondly, the formulation of and actions taken within the legal framework of governance should be characterised by *rule of law, transparency and accountability*. This implies respect of human rights and that all decision-makers are accountable for their actions. Finally, the third pillar is to ensure that governance is characterised by *equality, equity and efficiency*. This implies more substantive outcomes, in that "institutions and their processes should make the best use of resources to produce results that meet people's needs". Hsu exemplifies how HIV/AIDS applies to these governance ideals by posing three questions: Have men and women been taken into consideration equally when formulating HIV policies? Do HIV/AIDS-related laws and regulations uphold human rights and are they formulated and applied in a transparent way that allows for decision-makers to be held accountable? And, thirdly, have decisions on AIDS treatment respected the ideals of equality and equity?

The main argument in Hsu's analysis is that where the political response to the epidemic rests on the three pillars of democratic governance, societies are more HIV resilient; they are able to respond to a threatening epidemic in a way that prevents it from being unleashed in society or to react to an already established epidemic in a way that reduces incidence and generates effective treatment. By making inferences from some case studies, Hsu identifies five governance *mechanisms* that are critical in building such an HIV-resilient society (2004,: 5). (1) There has to be political *leadership with strategic vision* that unites all social and political sectors into a common effort that takes historical and cultural complexities into account. (2) Such a response has to be *timely*, ie the sooner it is launched the better. (3) The response also needs to be generated through *participation by civil society organisations*. Only when this sector plays a part throughout the whole process of policy formulation and implementation will the response benefit people in a sustainable way. (4) The response needs to be *multi-sectoral* in how it ties all government departments into a three-way partnership with civil society and the business sector. And finally (5) the response needs to be transparent and framed within institutions that make decision-makers *accountable* for their decisions.

Although the general points argued by Hsu seem reasonable and relevant, it is not clear on what basis they emerge from the empirical research included in the report, or in other words why these have proved to be decisive in generating a strong and effective response to the epidemic. The problem, arguably, is the way in which Hsu firstly designs and secondly reports the empirical research. Starting with the latter point, Hsu states simply that the different responses in Brazil, Uganda and Thailand approximated the ideals of democratic government and applied the mechanisms in their different policies. And yet, nowhere does she show explicitly that, for instance, accountability made an actual difference to how politicians chose to prioritise and respond for fear of sanctioning from the public in one form or another.

Likewise, nowhere is it made clear that activists or any other stakeholder made use of the information or strategic options that transparency offers to mobilise against an inactive government. What emerge instead from the three case studies is, arguably, how important it is for a society to be fortunate enough to have political leaders who respond wisely to the challenges of the epidemic. But that leaves us no wiser in terms of understanding and advocating governance issues in relation to the epidemic where such leadership is lacking. A related methodological problem with Hsu's empirical research is that all cases referred to are successful cases in one sense or another: prevalence levels have remained low in Thailand through early and strong prevention campaigns and prevalence has been reduced and treatment programmes are relatively efficient in both Uganda and Brazil. Clearly, if we wish to understand why some characteristics of political responses to HIV/AIDS have been more efficient than others, we need to also analyse the experiences in countries that have failed in dealing with the epidemic despite much effort.

One case in point is Botswana, a country to which most if not all of the generalisations that Hsu generates apply and yet prevalence levels there have been rising, despite such interventions to a point where they are now the highest in the world. Methodologically, Hsu's empirical research is erroneously designed and does not sustain the generalisations she makes. This does not mean that she is necessarily wrong in what she says or suggests, but that the report does not provide the systematic empirical research needed to back up her argument.

Finally, an additional problem with Hsu's argument is that she suggests that the more a response is characterised by democracy – in terms of participation, human rights and accountability – the better and stronger the response is. Nowhere does she really reflect on the internal tensions and inherent dilemmas of such a democratic response. One is led to believe that the philosophical, theoretical and practical problems that result from conflicting ideals within the democratic paradigm are irrelevant for democratic governance; but unfortunately not all good things go together. *Participation* is costly and will reduce the speed with which the government can respond. While some participation is likely to increase legitimacy and improve the sustainability of the political intervention, it does not in itself guarantee high quality or a particular character of the response. And what if the majority of participants or those most resourceful insist on a moral crusade against the epidemic, arguing that those affected are rightfully paying the price for their sinful behaviours? Such an unfortunate approach would be impossible if the response builds on human rights, as defined by the 1948 United Nations Declaration of Human Rights.

However, to proscribe a *human rights* approach is no panacea against difficult decisions. It does not, for instance, resolve whether the emphasis should be put on the HIV-positive individual's right to secrecy and integrity or on the non-infected individual's right to protection from potential infection; the dilemma at the centre of debates on the wisdom of making HIV a notifiable disease. Finally, to the extent that *accountability* in this context is taken to mean the electorates' ability to vote politicians out of office for what they did or did not do in response to the epidemic, this is a double-edged sword for advocates of democratic governance. As was discussed in chapter two, in the harsh political context of governments in less than consolidated democracies that are having to fight basic poverty-related problems, democratic accountability might see responsible and committed governments with viable but unpopular policies for countering complex and long-term effects of the epidemic being voted out of office in favour of populist political entrepreneurs whose ill-conceived responses are attractive to poorly educated and/or prejudiced electorates.

While democracy trumps all alternative political regimes, it cannot be assumed to generate good policy or effective implementation always, certainly not in the context of the HIV/AIDS epidemic. The question then is how we can improve on the chances of it doing just that; generating a strong and effective response to the epidemic. One avenue to pursue in researching this aspect of democratic governance would be to look at creating institutional incentives that counter those facets of the democratic process which, in the context of the epidemic, are less attractive. As a first take on such a discussion, our next section suggests a list of democratic governance principles that, arguably, ought to guide the formulation of policy on HIV/AIDS.

3.2.5 ADVOCATING DEMOCRATIC GOVERNANCE ON HIV/AIDS

At the end of this section we shall make a specific contribution to the advocacy of democratic governance on HIV/AIDS, but first we need to review a recent international initiative that seeks to set the norms for how governments should act in response to the epidemic. Following the United Nations General Assembly Special Session (UNGASS) on HIV/AIDS held in 2001 and the identification of specific goals in reducing the prevalence of AIDS as part of the UN's Millennium Goals,[9] the UN's *Commission on HIV/AIDS and Governance in Africa* was launched in 2003 to consider the long-term impact of the epidemic in Africa and make recommendations to the UN Secretary-General Kofi Annan by June 2005. At a recent conference in Ethiopia the commission presented what it called a "synopsis" of that forthcoming report (ECA, 2004). Good governance, writes the ECA, in the introduction to its synopsis:

> *is at the heart of sustainable development and the alleviation of poverty. It clearly is good for economic growth. It augments production inputs, such as labour and capital, and enhances the productivity of those inputs. It can also influence the distribution of benefits of economic growth: income distribution is a crucial factor in transforming growth into poverty reduction in Africa. Governance thus has a dual impact: on growth and its distribution. So better governance, by increasing growth and improving income equity, can reduce poverty and spur advances towards the Millennium Goals (Ibid: 9).*

The quote seems to represent a bias in the analytical framework towards an economic analysis of governance, but this is balanced in other sections of the report that emphasise the need for interventions against corruption and other mismanagement by strengthening different organs of the state, such as the judiciary and the bureaucracy. A particularly interesting section addresses the need to make constructive use of traditional leadership structures in the realisation of good governance. Taking into account that the report is not a finished product and that the thinking of the ECA is presented in brief it is nevertheless noteworthy that its section on how to respond to the HIV/AIDS epidemic is quite weak on practical suggestions and critical interventions, especially in terms of how to strengthen democratic governance as a response to the epidemic. Some additional suggestions are mentioned in the *Consensus Statement* that was issued at the conference, but there is arguably a need to reformulate the proposals on good governance through the prism of a more critical and politically forthright analytical framework if the proposals are to have a real effect, given the problematic experiences of governance failures on the continent.

Our own suggestions in this section in terms of advocacy for stronger democratic governance on HIV/AIDS are elaborations and specifications of the list of nine principles of democratic governance that are formulated by the UNDP in its *Human Development Report* of 2002. The UNDP's more general principles are listed as UNDP 1-9, and our contributions as IDASA 1-9:

UNDP 1: *People's human rights and fundamental freedoms are respected, allowing them to live with dignity.*

IDASA 1: A balance must be struck that respects the rights of those who are infected, as well as the rights of those who are not. The individual's rights to secrecy about his/her HIV status and treatment against AIDS are as fundamental as his/her right to protection from HIV. Any political intervention that imposes on any of these rights must be legitimised through public deliberation and due legal process.

UNDP 2: *People have a say in decisions that affect their lives.*

IDASA 2: Policies on HIV/AIDS must be formulated and debated in a transparent process that allows people living with AIDS and other stakeholders extra opportunity for participation and influence. At the very least the opportunity for people to choose between alternative political interventions as proposed by contending parties in free and fair elections is paramount.

UNDP 3: *People can hold decision-makers accountable.*

IDASA 3: Where decision-makers fail to fulfil promises or implement inefficient policies in the fight against HIV/AIDS, those ultimately responsible must accept to stand down if their (in)actions have undermined their credibility in the eyes of the stakeholders or the public in general. A number of institutional arrangements can affect such accountability, of which free and fair democratic elections is the most common.

UNDP 4: *Inclusive and fair rules, institutions and practices govern social interactions.*

IDASA 4: Inclusive and fair rules, institutions and practices govern social interactions between those who are and those who are not infected and/or directly affected by HIV and AIDS.

UNDP 5: *Women are equal partners with men in private and public spheres of life and decision-making.*

IDASA 5: Due to being particularly vulnerable to the epidemic, women's experiences of being directly or indirectly affected by the epidemic must be prioritised in all decision-making.

UNDP 6: *People are free from discrimination based on race, ethnicity, class, gender or any other attribute.*

IDASA 6: HIV/AIDS is of no lesser concern or importance to society as a whole if it mainly affects one or more population segment that is relatively marginalised from power. As a means to reduce the stigma attached to HIV/AIDS, the right to non-discrimination for those living with the virus should be elevated to the same level as other fundamental rights given to other categories of the population.

UNDP 7: *The needs of future generations are reflected in current practices.*

IDASA 7: The different decisions on prioritisation of resources and rights that go into formulating HIV/AIDS policy must take into consideration also the needs of today's AIDS orphans and the sustainability of society beyond their generation.

UNDP 8: *Economic and social policies are responsive to people's needs and aspirations.*

IDASA 8: Government policy on HIV/AIDS must adapt in accordance with perceived incidence and estimated prevalence of HIV and experienced illnesses and deaths from AIDS.

UNDP 9: *Economic and social policies aim at eradicating poverty and expanding the choices that all people have in their lives.*

IDASA 9: Government policy on HIV/AIDS also must address the structural problems that impact on the prevalence of HIV and reduce the receptiveness in people to treatment against AIDS. Only a person who has both information and realistic alternatives is truly empowered to change a behaviour that fuels the epidemic.

This initial formulation of what would constitute democratic governance in relation to HIV/AIDS highlights the particular importance of one fundamental democratic institution – free and fair elections. Although holding elections is not sufficient for a regime to qualify as a democracy, the institution represents one of the most basic and important aspects of democracy: the peaceful and legitimate replacement of people in positions of power. The electoral process – by which the people choose among candidates and elect those vested with the power to make laws on their behalf – is perhaps the most central of democratic processes. Like few others it realises some of the core principles of democracy: equal citizenship, freedom of opinion and accountability. Indeed, the point of listing the nine principles above can be restated as the definition of the nine grounds on which a government might lose power because of its failures in dealing with the HIV/AIDS epidemic. But such failure need not be due to a lack of commitment from the government. In fact, and ironically, it can be the result of the destructive impact that the epidemic has had on the capacity of the state and its democratic processes.

3.3 HOW IS HIV/AIDS A THREAT TO DEMOCRATIC GOVERNANCE?

When we turn the question around from asking how different political responses might impact on the epidemic and ask how the epidemic affects governance, we find ourselves in a literature that mainly consists of scholarly hypotheses. There are as yet few empirical analyses that can point to clear results on this issue. But before we review some of these debates we briefly need to contextualise our inquiry in the problematic experiences of governance in Africa more generally. While the epidemic is the most recent and alarming threat to governance in Africa (Fortin, 1990; Hunter, 2003), poor governance has a long history on the continent.

3.3.1 DEMOCRATIC GOVERNANCE IN AFRICA

With a few notable exceptions, the effort to realise democratic governance in Africa is not yet 15 years old. We should therefore not expect too much as none of the presently consolidated democracies in Europe and America had met the criteria for democratic governance that we saw above in such a short time after formally becoming democratic, decades or centuries ago. However, the main problem is not that time has been short, but that in this short space of time many of the political systems seem to have drifted further away from the ideals of democratic governance. Scholars have given different names to this complex political problem, of which "neopatrimonialism" is most common. With its origins in the sociology of Max Weber, the concept should be understood as capturing the problematic political dynamic that results from the mismatch between a formal political system and state bureaucracy that is structured according to a "modern" institutional order, and an informal "patrimonial" set of norms that govern how power is actually legitimised and used. The problematic features of neopatrimonialism have been identified as corruption, the personalisation of power and *clientilism* (Bratton & De Walle, 1997).

When the empirical criteria for good governance that Hyden suggested above are applied to a political system dominated by neopatrimonialism, one finds, firstly, that "the degree to which citizens can have influence and oversight of the political process" is restricted. Corruption has often blurred any transparency and undermined the concept of the rule of law to the point that the bribe has surpassed the vote as a means to influence government. Secondly, "the degree to which leadership is responsive and responsible" is low since leaders have personalised power and show responsiveness mainly to the *clientilistic* network that maintains them in power. Personalised power also is centralised power; no other institution or social sphere is granted autonomous power that in any substantial way can check the personal ambitions of the ruler. Thirdly, and consequently, "the degree to which interactions in civil society are characterised by social reciprocities" will be low since people in civil society will have no incentives to live and organise according to such reciprocities when the formal political system is defined by corruption, *clientilism* and the abuse of power. Neopatrimonialism will tend to dissolve the generalised social trust that is necessary for social reciprocities and block incentives for collective action in civil society.

While this account of the problems with governance in Africa is valid as a very general description, it gives a skewed reflection of realities on at least two accounts that are particularly relevant for our inquiry. The South African democracy and state does not suffer from these problems on the scale that the general account suggests. While there have been individual cases of corruption, and while some government bureaucracies are particularly affected, the problem is not as severe as in other countries in Africa. What is even more important is that corruption in South Africa is not accepted as an informal code of practice. Much energy and resources are spent in fighting the problem and people in high offices have resigned after being sanctioned by the courts. The second important deviation is that much is being done to improve democratic governance at a regional and African level. An important element to the African Renaissance – the fight against different forms of corruption and other practices of bad governance – is high on the agenda of both the Southern African Development Cooperation (SADC) and the African Union (AU).

These nuances notwithstanding, the concept of neopatrimonialism is arguably still relevant as an analytical tool for understanding general problems with democratic governance in Africa. By briefly establishing a link between the two concepts we can see that, as a general characterisation, African political systems fell short of good governance for some time before they had to face the additional problem of HIV/AIDS on their resources and institutions of governance. With the introduction of the more qualitatively demanding concept of "democratic governance" in 2002 – at a time when countries had started to really feel the effects of AIDS – the ambition to not only subscribe to democratic governance principles in general but also in political practice has become considerably more difficult. But what is it in more detail that the epidemic does to undermine the democratic, political and bureaucratic processes of the African state? The literature can present few certainties, but a number of plausible and worrying hypotheses.

3.3.2 THE IMPACT OF HIV/AIDS ON GOVERNANCE

One can speak of two more general ways in which the epidemic presents problems for governance in Africa: it undermines capacity to put good governance into practice and it alters the rationale for political and social action by individuals and communities.

REDUCED CAPACITY FOR DEMOCRATIC GOVERNANCE

As we saw in the previous chapter, the people most at risk of infection are those in the most sexually active ages of between 15 and 49, an age bracket that also captures people's most active years in their professional lives. A great majority of teachers, nurses, civil servants and workers of all trades will be found in that age cohort. If these people cannot access sustainable antiretroviral (ARV) treatment, we are going to see a considerable reduction in numbers due to AIDS-related illness and premature death, an impact that will quickly aggregate to a reduction in the capacity of the state to provide necessary services and economic growth. This impact is compounded by the lack of skilled and highly skilled workers in the South African labour force. As noted by Nattrass (2004: 150-154) even a relatively small impact of the epidemic on this category of workers will have a noticeable macroeconomic effect as there is virtually no unemployment among them, ie there is no one to replace those who have to leave their careers prematurely, resulting in a problematic skills shortage. And further, since this group of skilled and highly skilled workers also emigrate in considerable numbers, it is crucial that those who are HIV positive among them have access to the necessary treatment that as far as possible enables them to pursue "normal" life-long careers.

Apart from trying to predict the impact of this loss of professional skills, scholars have tried also to estimate the loss of capacity for good governance in financial terms. However, the question *what is the macroeconomic impact of AIDS?* is not easy to answer (Lewis 2004). After reviewing the various more authoritative attempts at modelling this impact in the literature, Nattrass concludes that one is left in "a rather confused state, to say the least" (Nattras, 2004: 160). Since different groups of researchers use different theoretical and behavioural assumptions in their respective models they reach different conclusions. Nattrass concludes: "One must be very cautious about all macroeconomic models of the impact of AIDS. At best they help us think through the dynamic economic impact of AIDS. At worst, they are a misleading and shaky house of cards" (Nattrass, 2004: 162). Keeping this advice in mind we can discern two general scenarios in the literature, one less pessimistic and one very pessimistic.

The general argument in the less pessimistic scenario is that while GDP growth will be reduced by 0.6 percentage points a year (for the years 2002-2015), per capita income will still rise as AIDS will reduce the population growth at a higher rate than it impacts negatively on GDP growth. Similarly, while the rate of employment falls, the total rate of unemployment will still be lowered as the labour force is reduced faster than the demand for labour. This scenario is one where the horrendous impact of the epidemic on those humans and communities who are directly and severely affected is offset by positive economic trends for those who are not similarly affected, either because they are not infected or because they have access to the medication that allows them to lead next-to-normal lives. The aggregate impact on the state's capacity in this scenario consequently would be less problematic; the loss of some human capital would to a considerable extent be compensated for by increased opportunities and capacities for others.

In the more pessimistic scenario, on the other hand, the state's capacity would be undermined considerably with a reduced growth of two percentage points a year (for the years 2002-2010), a drop that would be greater than the reduced population growth, leading to an overall reduction in per capita income. These projections, coupled with a steady unemployment rate, leads to the conclusions that, different from the less pessimistic model above, "the survivors of the AIDS epidemic are left with a smaller economic 'pie' and more of this pie is directed towards non-discretionary health and food expenditures" (Arndt & Lewis, 2000: 879-881, cited in Nattrass, 2004: 160). Clearly, in this scenario, the aggregate effect would be a loss of capacity for good governance in the state, partly as a result of a shortage of labour and skills and partly as a result of less financial resources with which to realise policies of state-led development. But we shall see that the impact is likely to go beyond the loss of skills and labour and financial margins as we now turn to explore hypothesised effects of state institutions and political behaviour more generally.

NEW RATIONALE FOR POLITICAL AND SOCIAL ACTION

Many hypotheses in the emerging social science literature about the destructive effects of the epidemic for governance build on the realisation that previous assumptions of individual rationality are no longer relevant since people are likely to die sooner and face additional hardships for themselves and their families than what was the case before the epidemic. As a consequence of this, people will change their social and political behaviours to accommodate these new circumstances. Alex de Waal discusses the implications of the shorter life span and loss of human resources and skills for governance within state institutions and argues that:

> *Complex modern institutions are framed around decades-long working lives. The running of a bureaucracy such as a ministry, a large firm or an army depends on staff who have not only the professional skill but also many years of experience and extensive networks and personal contacts ... No training course or rule-book can substitute for the experience, contacts and judgement that accrue over a lifetime career. ... Reduced life expectancy on attaining adulthood, coupled with the increased need for immediate medical expenditure, also distorts the structure of incentives and deterrents for opportunistic or corrupt behaviour. Instead of 25 years to build a house to provide for one's dependants, a civil servant may believe he/she has only five or ten years. ... The longer-term institutional impact follows from the sustained nature of these problems: the losses are not a one-off shock to the system. (2003:11-12).*

On the basis of this logic we would expect an increased level of corruption as a consequence of the epidemic. While the hypothesis might hold true for individual institutions in the southern African countries, explorative research shows that there is not yet a discernable pattern of increased corruption, as measured by

Transparency International, in countries in the region where HIV prevalence is particularly high or has risen sharply in the past few years (Wisten, forthcoming).

If we expand the discussion and relate it to the notion of democratic governance, the problems are compounded even further. Jeremy Youde elaborates on three aspects of the threat that the epidemic poses to the stability and legitimacy of democracy in sub-Saharan Africa. Democratic regimes might become illegitimate if the electoral processes by which they are elected are undermined by the epidemic as "burdensome voter registration requirements and the loss of skilled, non-partisan bureaucrats to supervise elections will threaten the impartial administration of elections and make electoral fraud more likely" (Youde, forthcoming: 6). Secondly, in line with our review above, the epidemic also will undermine the chances for successful democratisation as the economy is likely to suffer from the loss of skills and labour to AIDS-related illnesses and deaths. And thirdly, the increased morbidity and mortality will reduce the strength and sustainability of the constructive challenge that civil society can mobilise against the state and political parties. (Youde, forthcoming: 6).

Concurring with Youde, Bob Mattes elaborates further on some of these points in an overview article (2003:6-11). According to Mattes' reasoning, the epidemic is likely to affect the democracies in the region by undermining the institutions, changing the political attitudes of voters and increasing prejudice and intolerance in civil society. On the institutional level HIV/AIDS risks undermining democratic elections since the fair and legitimate administration of the electoral process is going to be more problematic. With increasing numbers of potential voters severely ill from AIDS, a great number of eligible voters face disenfranchisement if the electoral administration does not have the capacity to make special arrangements for them to register and vote. The greatly increased death rate also will undermine the accuracy of the voters' roll, thus enabling governments to use "ghost voters" to their benefit. These effects will combine in undermining the legitimacy of the elections since they will be less fair than they otherwise would have been.

The other institutional effect concerns the loss of human skills and experiences in the elected representative bodies at all levels of government. In this respect, however, a rapid turnover of people due to AIDS deaths represents a greater loss than in other organisations. A political career is more than skills and experience. It represents – hopefully – the accumulation of trust and legitimacy between the politician and both people in general and his/her colleagues in the legislature and/or government. Such personal qualities are never automatically transferred to the person who is appointed or elected to replace the deceased politician. The overall effect of this loss will differ depending on what electoral system is used, as is discussed further in chapter four below.

Citizens' attitudes in relation to democracy also might be adversely affected by HIV/AIDS. If democratic governments are or seem to be unable to deal with the crisis, people might – in the worst case scenario – turn to just about any politician who promises forceful action against the epidemic. Such a development would open the door for authoritarian political entrepreneurs with simple answers to complex problems. People might end up participating less in politics also as this appears meaningless and resources are better spent caring for sick members of the family or community.

Finally, writes Mattes, the epidemic might generate and provide an outlet to values and norms in civil society that run counter to democracy as such and particularly to the liberal democratic notion of a tolerant and empowering civil society functioning as a "school of democracy" for people in general. The likely combination of populism and, in Mattes terminology, an "uncivil" society is likely to cause an additional counter-intuitive political dynamic with a problematic potential. A critical moment for a government in a developmental context severely affected by AIDS will be "*after* it becomes affordable to provide antiretroviral treatment to some employees and citizens, but *before* it becomes possible to provide them to all" (Mattes, 2003: 9-10). Just as has been the case in for example Zimbabwe with politically biased government-controlled food distribution in the context of starvation, any perception that political expediency determines who gets treatment and who does not could rapidly mobilise people for political turmoil. "Thus", Mattes concludes, "political decisions around AIDS treatment hold the potential to aggravate tensions and political conflict between workers and unemployed, urban and rural populations, or between different ethnic groups" (Mattes, 2003: 9-10).

Although it lies outside the actual focus of this research project, we also need to mention the research that suggests that democratic governance might not only deteriorate as a consequence of the epidemic, but that it might be done away with altogether through armed conflict (Ostergaard, 2002). It has long been obvious that armed conflicts increase the spread of the virus through the sexual violence of invading soldiers and the forced and rapid disintegration of social norms and networks as large numbers of people are forced to flee to avoid death in the fighting (Elbe, 2002). But the causal link is turned the other way with the argument that the level of insecurity and risk of war increases when the capacity and effectiveness of military armies are undermined by shockingly high rates of HIV prevalence that, in turn, represent the "security vacuum" that can be exploited by political entrepreneurs with a military strategy who might launch military initiatives that they otherwise would have refrained from had the opposing army been in good health and at full capacity (Schönteich and Pharaoh, 2003). This problematic scenario is arguably relevant only where levels of insecurity between states and/or insurgent armies are already high. AIDS will not cause wars on its own, but it might contribute to the outbreak of conflict – and thus the complete demise of democratic governance – where sick armies are no longer effective deterrents.

CONCLUDING REMARKS

The horrible scenario of HIV prevention programmes and AIDS treatment drugs becoming part of the patronage used by incumbents to hold on to power arguably borders on being apocalyptic. This is not an African reality today and very little suggests that it will ever become the reality in South Africa. Such a scenario would be placed at the extreme end of the governance spectrum that places democratic governance on HIV/AIDS at the opposite end. Irrespective of our opinion of the likelihood of African governments intentionally reducing governance on HIV/AIDS to anything that even approximates the apocalypse, we can probably agree on the importance of identifying democratic governance as the all-important ideal. However, as our discussion has tried to emphasise, we do the advocacy and prospects for success of such governance a great disservice if we shy away from its problematic aspects and inherent dilemmas. Only by critically exploring ways of reducing its weaknesses can we improve on the mechanisms of democratic governance to generate effective responses to the epidemic. While much can be done in terms of institutionalising political incentives for politicians to act upon, the political pressure for such reforms must originate ideally in civil society to gain full legitimacy.

Part 2

Exploring the Impact of HIV & AIDS on Central Electoral Institutions

We should perhaps remind ourselves that this topic is not the subject of academic curiosity only. High level politicians have begun recently to voice their concerns about AIDS-induced by-elections.

Chapter 4

Impact of HIV/AIDS on Electoral Systems

Much of the policy and academic discourse on HIV/AIDS has revolved around the implications and impact of the epidemic on socioeconomic development, most of which concludes that HIV/AIDS is developmental catastrophe. All the UNAIDS global reports on the epidemic unequivocally point to this stark reality of our times. The analysis in this chapter introduces an alternative set of complexities and impacts with direct links to how the epidemic undermines democratic governance more generally and how the epidemic affects the legitimacy and sustainability of electoral systems in southern Africa in general and South Africa in particular. The chapter will highlight the significance of elections and electoral systems to a working democracy and suggest that the impact of HIV/AIDS on governance is likely to vary from country to country depending on the nature of the electoral system in place.

We should perhaps remind ourselves that this topic is not the subject of academic curiosity only. High level politicians have begun recently to voice their concerns about AIDS-induced by-elections. At the African Development Forum(ADF) held at Addis Ababa, Ethiopia, in October 2004 by the Economic Commission for Africa (ECA) and the African Union(AU), the leader of the opposition in the Malawian parliament, Mr John Tembo, responded to an anecdotal presentation of IDASA's work by the United Nations Commission on AIDS and Governance by seeking solutions to this very phenomena: AIDS is apparently causing too many by-elections, he said. What must we do about it? Must we stop people who are infected from seeking office? Similarly, in a submission to a special committee set up to review the electoral law in Zambia, former Finance Minister Dr Katele Kalumba, posed a fundamental question: had the state considered what would happen if it lost a president within a few months of electing him/her given the huge costs that go into the polls? Would the budget sustain a presidential by-election?

In short what we discuss here is already a source of debate. There is awareness that this problem is inherent and needs attention. It also underlines the linkage between the disease and the electoral model, which we shall illustrate henceforth.

The link between the HIV/AIDS epidemic and electoral systems essentially revolves around the various challenges posed by having to fill an increasing number of vacant seats in elected assemblies in mid-term due to the AIDS-related illnesses and deaths of elected representatives. In countries that operate the so called First-Past-The-Post (FPTP) electoral system, such as Zambia, Lesotho and Zimbabwe, elected representatives can be replaced only through by-elections in their respective constituencies, a process that drains already strained state coffers. In the alternative Proportional Representation (PR) system, used for instance in South Africa and Namibia, vacant seats are filled not through elections but by the affected party appointing a member according to his/her ranking on a list of candidates. In some countries the two systems might be combined into hybrid versions of one type or another. While PR dominates the South African system, for example, some councillors in local government are elected according to the FPTP system, necessitating by-elections for their replacement in case of severe illness or death. In elaborating this general implication of the epidemic on electoral systems, this chapter will focus on the following four points:

- The process of holding by-elections imposes considerable financial costs that, in the context of the HIV/AIDS epidemic in southern Africa, threaten the mid- to long-term sustainability of FPTP electoral systems;
- The replacement of elected representatives amounts in most instances to a substantial political cost for the affected party, as well as the political system as a whole, irrespective of type of electoral system, due to the loss of experience, leadership and trust of the voters;
- The replacement of elected representatives through by-elections might incrementally alter power-relations in legislative assemblies to the point that the party which in the most recent election was entrusted with forming the government might see its parliamentary base undermined, thus making the legislative and other governance processes more difficult; and
- Since by-elections often attract lower voter participation than do national elections, the representatives thus elected hold weaker mandates in terms of constituency representation.

We start with a broader discussion on the significance of elections and electoral systems for democratic governance before we zero in on the impact of HIV/AIDS on the electoral system.

4.1 ELECTIONS AND ELECTORAL SYSTEMS

A democratic election is the process through which citizens choose their political representatives in legislative assemblies and, in some democratic systems, who should be the president of the country. While holding elections is not sufficient for qualifying as a democracy, no country can be a democracy without such elections (Nohlen, 1984:11). As the institutional process that transfers the citizens' political ideas and priorities into seats in the legislative assemblies, the legitimacy of the democratic system as such depends to a large degree on the "freeness and fairness" of elections. Elections are, in that sense, one of the most important features of a democracy.

The different rules that determine the nature and process of elections and how, more precisely, citizens' votes are transferred into seats in legislative assemblies comprise the electoral system of a particular country. While the core principle of that system – whether it is majoritarian such as the single member plurality system or First-Past-the-Post (FPTP) or Proportional Representation (PR) – is usually set out in a country's constitution and its many details are regulated in ordinary legislation (the electoral law). The central distinction between the electoral law and the electoral system has been formulated thus:

> *While electoral law determines the procedures to be adopted for the actual conduct of elections (secret ballot, counting of votes, impersonation, postal ballots and so on), the electoral system determines the way in which votes are cast and the relationship between votes and the allocation of seats. In*

> *other words, an electoral system is a method converting votes cast by electors into seats in the legislature. Electoral systems thus are the practical instruments through which notions such as consent and representation are translated into reality (Asmal and de Ville, 1994:1-2).*

It is important to note that these institutional arrangements not only create a government with a mandate to rule, but also a parliamentary opposition with an obligation to represent dissenting views and present alternative policies. Elections and electoral systems are no less than the rules and regulations through which conflicting parties and interests have agreed to settle their disputes over political power by peaceful means. As we briefly review the South African electoral system below, we shall note how central it was for the successful democratic transition in South Africa that the parties could agree on the principles for an electoral system at an early stage in the process.

One can speak of six ideal features of an electoral system (Krennerich and Nohlen, 1998:56-57). No existing system gets a full score on all these features; they rather emphasise some features over others. A system should allow parliament to be *representative* of a plurality of different interests in society by also enabling relatively small minority parties to win seats. This is a basic criterion for democracy to succeed in ethnically heterogeneous societies where minority groups otherwise might choose to pursue an armed conflict to secure their interests. However, to counteract the risk of too many parties making the assembly ineffective as a legislative institution, the system should seek to *concentrate* the political system on addressing the issues that most people prioritise. A system should give incentives for high levels of *participation* from the voters by avoiding procedures and requirements that are too costly in time and other resources for the individual voter. An electoral system also should ensure *accountability* in that voters can identify how an individual representative or a political party has handled the mandate given to them in the last election and reward or sanction them accordingly in the next election. A further feature is that a system should be as *simple* and transparent as possible so that it is well understood by the voters, a quality that will increase participation in elections, as well as reduce the number of spoilt votes. Finally, as a more general feature, an electoral system has to be regarded as *legitimate* by the voters and contending parties to sustain the democratic system over time..

It is clear that an electoral system is not "neutral" but different alternative principles and finer institutional mechanisms will make it more likely that some representatives are chosen over others, will allow some political ideals to dominate over others and will ensure that political power takes on some particular characteristics. We shall exemplify below what these variations might be, but our concluding point here is that an electoral system, as well as the elections to which it gives structure, are both finely tuned democratic instruments that in many ways epitomises the ideal of "government by the people". If, for whatever reason, they are seen not to be legitimate, not free and not fair, this will affect the sustainability of the whole democratic system and form of government. There is no general agreement in the international academic literature on what system is best for ensuring democratic governance and political stability (see for instance de Ville and Steytler, 1996; Sisk and Reynolds, 1998; Harris and Reilly, 1998; Reynolds and Reilly, 2002; Konrad-Adenauer-Stiftung, 2003). While most would agree that no system is best for all types of societies, scholars differ in what they suggest for different societies and there is much detail in the finer mechanics of electoral systems over which to argue. What none of these experts has considered, so far, in the calculation on what is the ideal electoral system for a particular society is what impact the HIV/AIDS epidemic will have on the society in general and the electoral process in particular. Further below we shall present some empirical information from southern Africa that we argue should motivate the consideration of the HIV/AIDS epidemic in the design of electoral systems.

4.1.1 Basic elements of electoral systems in southern Africa

Both of the two main types of electoral systems – the FPTP and PR systems – are represented among the democracies in southern Africa. Among the countries that use the FPTP electoral system are Botswana, Malawi, Swaziland, the Seychelles, Tanzania, Zambia and Zimbabwe, a majority of which are former British colonies. The PR system is used in Angola, Mozambique, Namibia and South Africa, while Lesotho and Mauritius recently have adopted the hybrid Mixed Member Proportional Representation (MMP) system (Matlosa, 2003a; Matlosa 2003b).

The FPTP system

The FPTP electoral system has a strong geographical component in that a country is divided into a great many distinct constituencies, each of which elects one representative to the legislative assembly. The number of constituencies corresponds exactly to the number of seats in parliament; save in situations where there are both elected and appointed members of parliament (as, for example, in Zimbabwe). Candidates contest elections within one of these constituencies either as representatives of a party or as independent candidates and the candidate who wins the most votes wins the right to represent the constituency; no absolute majority is necessary. The legitimacy of the FPTP system builds in many ways on the personal mandate that is given by the constituency to the successful candidate. While the candidate might (and often does) represent a political party, there is nevertheless an assumption that the candidate to some extent has a seat in parliament to protect the interests of all of the people in his/her "own" constituency. In some countries, the constituency has the right, under certain conditions, to "recall" the mandate of the elected representative if it feels misrepresented. While this strong personal tie between the constituency and its representative has many positive features, it implies that a by-election has to be held if the representative who was elected in general elections has to resign or dies. It is, as we shall see below, this rather cumbersome requirement that makes the FPTP system vulnerable to the impact of the HIV/AIDS epidemic.

On a more general level, and based on the experiences of many countries, the FPTP system can be said to give the following characteristics to the democratic system. Over time the system is likely to generate a two-party system (see below) as it favours large national parties at the exclusion of smaller and/or regional parties. A one-party government is likely to be formed by the largest party in the essentially two-party parliament. Such a government is less hindered in trying to realise its political programme and can be held accountable more easily for its successes and failures by the voters in the next election. This form of parliamentary set-up was a natural, and in many ways correct, reflection of political fault lines in England, its country of origin, at the time when industrialisation pitted representatives of capital against those of labour. But since the political realm is much more multi-dimensional in present-day countries, with people's political identifications determined not only by class but also by issues of gender, environment, culture and religion, the FPTP system is being challenged increasingly by demands for reforms to make it more sensitive to the concerns of minorities. Despite these shortcomings, the FPTP system has the advantage of being familiar to both voters and contending politicians in southern Africa.

THE LIST PR SYSTEM

Under the alternative PR system a country is either considered one large single constituency, or it is divided into a number of smaller voting districts, and more than one representative is elected from each district. The number of representatives from a district depends on the number of voters registered in that district and the contending parties gain representation from the district in proportion to its support among the voters. The representatives, however, do not have a personal mandate or a personal link to a particular district necessarily, but instead get elected to a legislative assembly on the basis of having been nominated internally by their party on to the list where it ranks its representatives; the more votes won by the party, the more of the people on the list get to take up a seat in the legislature. Thus, within the basic PR system, voters elect parties, not individual representatives. At a party conference prior to elections party members will have elected its representatives on to the list, but the party leadership nevertheless has the final say on the composition and ranking of the lists. While this places much power in the hands of the party elite, a power that no doubt can be abused and corrupted to maintain networks of patronage and that is resistant to constructive change, it provides the opportunity to realise social and political goals such as equal gender representation in parliament and the representation of minorities of one kind or another. In the context of fighting the HIV/AIDS epidemic, party leaders could use this power over the lists to ensure that people with special knowledge and experience of the epidemic can make it on to the list and perhaps into legislative assemblies. We shall see in chapter six how this was attempted by one of the smaller parties that gained representation in the 2004 elections in South Africa.

Another important effect of the PR system is that parties can gain seats on the legislature even if they win only relatively few votes in the election. In some countries, for fear of the legislature becoming too divided and thus ineffective as a legislative institution, a threshold keeps parties out that do not gain, for instance, 4% of the vote. In other countries, South Africa being an example, there is no such formal threshold. The PR system is therefore more conducive for interest groups in civil society to make the transition successfully into a political party. In the context of fighting the HIV/AIDS epidemic it is therefore not unrealistic in any of the PR countries in southern Africa to expect the launch of a single-issue party that addresses the political response to the epidemic.

THE MMP SYSTEM

There are as many variations to these electoral systems as there are democratic states. One such variation, however, is identified as a third system in its own right: the Mixed Member Proportional (MMP) system. The MMP, in brief, aims to broaden representation (through a PR component) and retain accountability of elected representatives (through a FPTP component), thus seeking to strike a good balance between the two original systems. This is done by dividing the parliamentary seats so that some are won on a constituency vote and some are won on a party vote. On voting day the voter casts two votes, one for each section of parliament. The MMP system would thus be more conducive than the FPTP system for representing a small single-issue party or for allowing parties to nominate candidates who are particularly qualified to work with the issue of HIV/AIDS in the legislative process, but less so than a more straightforward PR system.

In concluding this section we restate our argument that the main concern when considering the impact of the epidemic on electoral systems is not how they differ in providing incentives for the issue of HIV/AIDS to gain representation in parliament, but rather what the implications are when an elected representative has to resign or dies while in office. Although elected representatives, at least on national and provincial levels, are likely to have access to some medical plan that enables them to receive ARV treatment, an increase in morbidity and mortality is already likely to have taken place that might increase even further in the future. It is in this perspective that the FPTP, and to a lesser degree, the MMPR systems are more vulnerable. Whereas in the PR system an elected representative is simply replaced by the next person on the party list, the FPTP system requires a by-election to be held in the affected constituency. We shall report further on the costs that are involved in such by-elections and discuss further implications for the democratic system as a whole.

4.2 THE SOUTH AFRICAN ELECTORAL SYSTEM

The current electoral model in use in South Africa since 1994 is the List-Proportional Representation system. According to Nohlen, a pure PR electoral system is one "which, without natural or artificial hurdles, (the size of constituencies or thresholds) aims at attaining the highest possible degree of proportionality" (cited in de Ville, 1996:19). Faure and Venter posit that "South Africa used the British FPTP system of electing representatives for parliament for more than 80 years. It remained essentially unchanged since its implementation of unification in 1910 until its replacement by a new electoral system with the 1993 Interim Constitution and the subsequent election of April 1994. Towards the end of the 1980s, it became clear that South Africa was irrevocably moving towards some major form of political transition and also a new electoral arrangement. The five years that preceded the adoption of the Interim Constitution in 1993 witnessed intensification in the debate on electoral options for the new South Africa" (2004:2). The following factors influenced South Africa's adoption of the PR model in 1994:

- Political compromise which was part of the 1990s political settlement;
- Imperatives for reconciliation, peace and harmony;
- Commitment towards nation-building and national unity by political protagonists who took part in the multiparty negotiations; and
- Desire to ensure broad political representation in parliament in a multiracial society following a centralised authoritarian system under the apartheid regime (see de Ville and Steytler, 1996).

However, the South African model is not as straightforward as it seems because the PR model applies only to elections for the national assembly. For local government elections the hybrid system that combines the constituency-based FPTP electoral model and PR is applied. The rationale for this was to ensure that at the national level there was a deliberate effort towards broadening representation in the national and provincial legislatures and nurturing and deepening reconciliation and political stability, while emphasis is placed upon accessibility and accountability at local government levels, even though in fact the FPTP system does tend to be exclusionary as indicated in the earlier sections of this chapter.

Under the British colonial administration and the apartheid regime South Africa used the FPTP electoral system. This system was changed in 1994 in line with the political changes that ushered in a democratic dispensation marked by majority rule and the demise of apartheid. The 1996 Constitution prescribes that the electoral system must result in general in proportional representation. Thus "the system chosen to fulfil this mandate for national parliament was a highly proportional party list system, in which each party draws up closed and rank-ordered national and provincial lists of candidates for parliament. Elections are held every five years" (Butler, 2004:105). Since 1994, therefore, South Africa has used the List-PR system in which the entire country is considered one big electoral zone or constituency with various voting districts. Parties contesting elections prepare lists of candidates for the 400-member national assembly as follows:

- A National Assembly list or national-to-national list comprising 200 candidates;
- A National Assembly list or province-to-national list comprising 200 candidates; and
- Nine provincial lists or provincial-to-province lists comprising candidates equivalent to the number of seats available in each provincial legislature (Cherry, 2004).

Having been duly constituted through an election, the national parliament "elects the president, who is the head of the executive branch of government, and who is responsible for governing in conjunction with the cabinet, which he appoints" (Butler, 2004:105). Thus, unlike in the FPTP system of the apartheid era, under the present PR electoral model, political parties prepare their party lists of candidates who in turn contest elections not as individuals chosen by the legislature to represent constituencies, but party representatives that essentially represent parties in the legislature. In terms of the seat allocation formula, (the so called "Droop quota"), the South African PR system provides for a fairly low threshold for parties' access to parliament compared with others in the SADC region, for example Mozambique (5%). The main purpose of a threshold is to determine inclusion and exclusion of parties in the legislature on the basis of votes cast per party contesting the elections. Thus, each party has to pass the test of implicit threshold first and foremost before gaining access to parliament.

It is worth emphasising, though, that the South African Constitution does not prescribe a predetermined or explicit threshold as such, given that this was perceived as undemocratic, exclusionary and discriminatory. Thus, the quota in South African elections is determined primarily by voter turn-out and the calculation of seats won by each party. Hence, according to Paul Graham, "the lower the voter turn-out, the lower the quota, thereby allowing more parties access to parliament; the higher the voter turn out, the higher the quota and the fewer the parties gaining parliamentary seats" (Interview, 19 August 2004). Essentially then in South Africa an implicit quota was considered a much more acceptable and democratic route to follow. Using the Droop method, "the quota of votes per seat (...) does, however, provide for an implicit threshold. The size of the implicit threshold is also dependent upon the way in which remaining seats are allocated, the number of votes cast and the number of spoilt papers" (De Ville, 1996:24). Corroborating De Ville, Faure and Venter aptly observe:

> *... for both the National Assembly and the regional/provincial legislatures the respective thresholds of various regions/provinces differ, unless they have the same numbers of seats in comparative cases. Approximately, 1/400th of votes cast for the national party lists of the National Assembly (ie about 0.25%) constitutes the threshold, but the number of seats already allocated regionally is subtracted from the seats won in this way, effectively making this threshold about 0.50%. The threshold for the National Assembly as a whole is 0.24938% (2003:5).*

The outcomes of the 1994, 1999 and 2004 elections were derived using this calculation culminating in the results as illustrated in table 10.

Table 10. Results in election to national assembly, 1994, 1999 and 2004

Election year	1994			1999			2004		
	Votes	Seats		Votes	Seats		Votes	Seats	
Party	%	actual	%	%	actual	%	%	actual	%
ANC	62.65	252	63.00	66.35	266	66.50	69.68	279	69.75
DP/DA	1.73	7	1.75	9.56	38	9.50	12.37	50	12.5
IFP	10.54	43	10.75	8.58	34	8.50	6.97	28	7
UDM	-	-	-	3.42	14	3.50	2.28	9	2.25
ID	-	-	-	-	-	-	1.73	7	1.75
NP/NNP	20.39	82	20.50	6.87	28	7.00	1.65	7	1.75
ACDP	0.45	2	0.50	1.43	6	1.50	1.6	6	1.5
FF/FF†	2.17	9	2.25	0.80	3	0.75	0.89	4	1
UCDP	-	-	-	0.78	3	0.75	0.75	3	0.75
PAC	1.25	5	1.25	0.71	3	0.75	0.73	3	0.75
FA	-	-	-	0.54	2	0.50	-	-	-
MF	-	-	-	0.30	1	0.25	0.35	2	0.5
Azapo	-	-	-	0.17	1	0.25	0.27	2	0.5

'-†-' indicates that the party did not participate or did not win a seat.
Source: The Independent Electoral Commission

It interesting to note how both the political opening brought about by the transition and the low threshold of the electoral model triggered a phenomenal mushrooming of political parties. However, despite the proliferation of parties, the three largest parliamentary parties on the national scene held 94% of the votes. The overwhelming support for the ANC has increased only in the two subsequent elections.

The ANC's electoral hegemony is firmly entrenched and the 2004 election result reinforces the dominant party system marked by an overwhelmingly strong ruling party on one hand and a fragmented opposition on the other. It has also held two local government elections in 1995 and 1999 and its third local government election since the 1994 political transition is scheduled for 2005.

Table 10 shows clearly how the PR system allots parliamentary seats to parties almost in direct proportion to their electoral strength; the percentage of votes a party won approximates were closely the number of seats it won in the National Assembly. This demonstrates the fairness and inclusivity of this system. Such strong correlation between the share of votes and seats is a rare or scarce political commodity under the FPTP system. While often criticised for the lack of accountability of MPs, given their strong link to the party rather than to the electorate, the PR system is regarded highly for its inherent values that seem to advance democratic governance, including broad representation of key political forces in the legislature, inclusivity of the political system, reconciliation in post-conflict societies and, equally importantly, gender balance in the governance realm as table 11 vividly demonstrates.

Table 11. Gender balance in the South African national assembly, 1994-2004

Year	Size of Parliament	Number of Women MPs	Women MPs in %
1994	400	111	27.7
1999	400	120	30.0
2004	400	131	32.7

Source: Morna, 2004; Gender Links website, 2004.

Women's participation in the South African parliament has increased steadily in the years since 1994. Women occupied 111 seats (or 27.7% of the total) out of a total of 400 seats in 1994. This representation increased by 8% to 120 seats in the 1999 election and by a further 9% in the 2004 elections. With a 32.8% of seats held by women, the South African parliament presently exceeds the goal set by the SADC Declaration on Gender and Development in 1997, to have 30% women representation in key organs of governance by the year 2005. There is no doubt that the electoral system has had an overbearing influence on this positive trend in South Africa's evolving democracy, but added to this has been commitment by political parties to inculcate a political culture that embraces gender equality in the governance process. However, what needs to be emphasised, though, is that the PR system on its own might not be an adequate catalyst for gender equality in the legislature. It needs additional impetus from political commitment to gender equality from the political elite in charge of party affairs and it also requires institutionalisation of either voluntary or involuntary quotas for women's representation in the legislature.

Having briefly reviewed the pattern of election results and the impact thereon of the electoral system in place in South Africa, it is worth noting that, directly or indirectly, the two variables (namely electoral contest and electoral system) have in a large measure also influenced the nature of the existing party system. As Lodge reminds us, "robust democracies benefit from strong parties. Strong parties attract durable support" (2004:189). A party system denotes procedures, rules and the institutional framework for the party political contest for state power within a given political system. The party system is, however, not confined merely to both inter-party and intra-party relations and how parties contest political power as such because it also extends to the articulation of party interests with interests and demands of popular organisations in society. According to the Encyclopaedia of Democracy, there are various characteristics of party systems including:

- Number of parties;
- Size of parties;
- Party political configuration in the national assembly;
- Party manifestos and programmes;
- Party relationships with interest/pressure groups (alliances);
- Inter-party relations; and
- Intra-party relations.

There are basically four types of party systems the world-over. namely (a) the one-party system that provides for a governance system in which only one party is in existence either *de jure* or *de facto* and actively drives the political system and is solely in control of state power; (b) a two-party system or *duopoly* wherein two main parties dominate and drive the political system and alternate over the control of state power through electoral contest; (c) a multi-party system in which more than two parties exist and are politically active in directing the governance realm and in so doing alternate the control over state power among themselves; and (d) the dominant party system in which, despite the multiparty situation, only one party is so dominant that it directs the political system and is firmly in control of state power over a fairly long duration of time so that even opposition parties make little, if any, dent on its political hegemony (Lodge, 2004; Karume, 2004). By all indications, therefore, the political hegemony of the ruling ANC suggests that the country's governance realm is marked by a dominant party system to all intents and purposes. Some of the key features of the dominant system, such as the one prevailing in South Africa, include:

- Continuous electoral victories of a dominant party over time by huge margins and as such reducing oppositional contest to second fiddle;
- Political hegemony of the ruling party over state institutions, including control of the largest share of the legislature and local government authorities; and
- Sole determination and direction of development policy trajectories by the ruling party with little challenge or credible policy alternatives from opposition parties over time.

We now turn the spotlight on the central subject of this chapter, the linkage between electoral system and HIV/AIDS.

4.3 How the epidemic impacts on electoral systems

In their recent literature survey on HIV/AIDS and governance in the SADC region, Kelly et al in responding to a question "what do we know?", argue persuasively that "the simple answer to the question… is that we know very little, because there is scarcity of substantive data and primary research on the topic of HIV/AIDS and democracy" (2002). Our aim with this section, therefore, is to contribute some original research and empirical findings to remedy this lack of research in the literature. Our discussion flows from four main strands of thought: (a) replacement of MPs becomes one of the major financial costs associated with elections especially in countries that operate the FPTP or MMP system due to the necessity of by-elections; (b) however, irrespective of whichever electoral system is in place, replacement of MPs in parliament amounts to a political cost for the party that loses members of the legislature; (c) replacement of MPs in parliament might have the effect also of shifting the power balance in the legislature often in favour of ruling parties and to the disadvantage of opposition parties; and (d) equally importantly, a related downside of by-elections under the FTPT or MMP system is that with low levels of voter turnout relative to national elections the political mandate of MPs gets technically denuded.

4.3.1 Costs associated with by-elections: Zambia and Zimbabwe

A recent study undertaken by IDASA in Zambia found that "the country's number of by-elections have substantially increased in the era of HIV/AIDS (1984-2003) compared with the 'Aids free era' (1964-1984)".

The pilot study undertaken in 2003 indicates that between 1964 and 1984 46 by-elections were held, only 14 of which were a result of death. While over an 18-year period (from 1985 to February 2003) 102 by-elections were held and 59 of those were due to death by disease. The majority of the 59, ie 39, were held between 1992 and February 2003, which coincidentally are the years in which the HIV/AIDS pandemic peaked in Zambia (Tapfumaneyi, 2003).

Table 12. By-elections in Zambia, 1964-2003

Years	Total number of by-elections held	By-elections held as a result of death	By-elections held as a result of resignations and expulsion
1964 to 1984	46	14 (30%)	32
1985 to 2003	102	59 (58%)	43

Source: Data from Electoral Commission and Zambia Parliament: A Statistical Profile 1964-1996.

While we do not know the cause of death of these MPs, we can make inferences that might help us with plausible conclusions. Firstly, the trends indicate a rise in the deaths of MPs in the period between 1985 (when the first case of HIV was documented) and 2003, and especially 1990-2003, which incidentally is the same phase in which HIV and AIDS peaked. Because of the absence of definitive indicators, we might glean something by examining the age brackets: do they fall within the 15-49 age range that is considered most vulnerable to HIV? The age range of those who passed away is as follows:

Table 13. Age cohort of deceased MPs, 1990-2003

Age cohort	30-39	40-49	50-59	60-69	70 +
Number of deceased MPs	0	15	12	9	2

Source: Idasa-GAP 2003.

The information is inconclusive at this stage and requires further research. There are though indications in the data that merit further research along the lines of our hypotheses above. The mere increase in mortality among Zambian MPs is in itself a change that needs an explanation. This trend might be particularly relevant in the context of the epidemic since 70% of the MPs who died between 1990 and 2003 would have been in their most sexually active phase during parts of that time period. However, the data need to be interrogated in further depth to provide a valid test to the hypothesis that HIV/AIDS is a possible explanation. We also need to state that we are aware that Zambia's parliament increased in size from 135 to 150 elective seats following the amendments to the constitutional/legal framework before the 1991 multiparty elections. There are also eight MPs nominated by the president of Zambia, but replacement of such MPs does not require by-elections.[10]

We need to underline, however, that it is not only the HIV/AIDS epidemic but any serious illness or cause of death that impose costs on countries running the FPTP system due to the holding of by-elections. If electoral processes on local level were to be included in the analyses we would be likely to see even more problematic trends.

The economic cost for Zambia for holding elections is substantial. Zambia has spent about $70 million on three national elections between 1991 and 2003. The 2001 tripartite polls consumed well in excess of $35 million (Chirambo, 2003:6; Chirambo, 2004:6).

Available evidence from the Zambia Electoral Commission suggests that the average cost for a by-election is $211 416 (Interview: Isaacs; 2004).[11] The 102 by-elections that were held between 1985 and 2003 thus amounted to roughly $21 600 000 at today's US dollar rate to the Zambian kwacha. The 59 by-elections due to death cost almost $12 500 000.

Thus, by-elections divert resources from the national budget, a problem that is compounded by the fact that they naturally are impossible to predict with any certainty. For this reason a majority of SADC states operating the FPTP system have tended to depend overwhelmingly upon donor support for their elections and this dependence is likely to deepen in the era of the HIV/AIDS epidemic. The trend of frequent costly by-elections under the FPTP electoral system in Zambia seems to be an all-pervasive phenomenon in the SADC countries operating this system, such as Zimbabwe and Lesotho (the latter despite its electoral reform of 2002). Since its parliamentary election in 2000 Zimbabwe has held 14 by-elections for the replacement of MPs as shown in table 14.

Table 14. By-elections in Zimbabwe, November 2000- May 2004

Constituency	Party that won 2000 election	Cause of MP replacement	Date of by-election	Party that won by-election
Marodera West	ZANU-PF	Illness	Nov. 2000	ZANU-PF
Bikita West	MDC	Illness	Jan. 2001	ZANU-PF
Bindura	ZANU-PF	Accident	July 2001	ZANU-PF
Makoni West	ZANU-PF	Accident	Sept. 2001	ZANU-PF
Chikomba	ZANU-PF	Illness	Sept. 2001	ZANU-PF
Inzisa	MDC	Illness	Oct. 2001	ZANU-PF
Highfield	MDC	Dismissal	Mar. 2003	MDC
Kuwadzana	MDC	Death	Mar. 2003	MDC
Makonde	ZANU-PF	Illness	Aug. 2003	ZANU-PF
Harare Central	MDC	Resignation	Aug. 2003	MDC
Kadoma Central	MDC	Illness	Nov. 2003	ZANU-PF
Gutu North	ZANU-PF	Illness	Feb. 2004	ZANU-PF
Zengeza	MDC	Resignation	Mar. 2004	ZANU-PF
Lupane	MDC	Illness	May 2004	ZANU-PF

Source: ZESN, Harare, Zimbabwe.

Although we are not able to establish the cost of general elections in Zimbabwe and that of by-elections, the frequency of these by-elections suggests that they place an onerous burden on the national budget. This also suggests that there is an urgent need for Zimbabwe, as there is for Zambia, to reform its electoral models more towards PR in full or at least the MMP system that Lesotho recently adopted and which Mauritius has decided to adopt in its forthcoming general election in 2005.

The data in the table above also speaks clearly to an additional implication of by-elections, a shift in power in the legislature. The general election in Zimbabwe in 2000 resulted in 62 elected seats for Zanu-PF, 57 elected seats for the opposition

Movement for Democratic Change (MDC) and one elected seat for Zanu-Ndonga. The political power balance in the legislature that was decided in the elections, however, changed gradually through a series of subsequent by-elections that increased the power for the ruling party. Since the 2000 election 13 by-elections have been held and another one is due to be held in due course. In this process the ruling Zanu-PF has gained by winning a majority of the by-elections and as such has increased its parliamentary strength from 62 to 67 seats, corresponding to the loss of parliamentary seats by the opposition MDC from 57 to 52 (see table 15).

Table 15. Power shift in parliament as a result of by-elections in Zimbabwe since the 2000 general election

Year	No of Seats			
Elections	ZANU-PF	MDC	ZANU Ndonga	Total
2000 General Election	62	57	1	120
By-Elections Since 2000*	67	52	1	120

*The MP for Seke constituency passed away over the weekend of 24th-25th July 2004. .Another by-election will therefore have to be held in this constituency before the parliamentary elections in March 2005. The date of the by-election is still to be arranged. Source: ZESN (Zimbabwe Election Support Network).

A fairly similar trend has been under way in neighbouring Zambia. As illustrated in table 4.7 below, since the 2001 general election, Zambia has had to replace 16 MPs so far due to a variety of factors, including resignations, expulsion, floor-crossing and nullification of results. In all the 16 cases the ruling MMD has been the main beneficiary in terms of increased seats in parliament, while the main opposition, the UPND, has been the main loser.

Table 16. Power shifts in parliament as result of replacement of MPs in Zambia since the 2001 general election

Constituency	Cause for MP replacement	Affected party	Party that gained due to replacement
Lufwanyama	Death	MMD	MMD
Bwacha	Defection	HP	MMD
Kabwe Central	Defection	HP	MMD
Mwandi	Expulsion	UPND	MMD
Keembe	Death	MMD	MMD
Mwansabombwe	Death	MMD	MMD
Nangoma	Resignation	UPND	MMD
Kantanshi	Death	MMD	PF
Solwezi Central	Resignation	UPND	MMD
Kaoma Central	Resignation	UPND	MMD
Lukulu East	Nullified	UPND	MMD
Msanzala	Nullified	UNIP	MMD
Mulobezi	Nullified	MMD	MMD
Mpika Centrakl	Nullified	MMD	MMD
Mwaninilunga East	Defection	UPND	MMD
Kantashi	Death	PF	PF

Source: Foundation for Democratic Process (FODEP)

4.3.2 COSTS ASSOCIATED WITH BY-ELECTIONS: LESOTHO

Most observers of Lesotho's political scene express a fair amount of optimism about the country's political prospects since the reform of its electoral model from the FPTP system to a MMP system (Elklit, 2003; Fox and Southall, 2003; Matlosa, 2004). Yet evidence suggests that this model might not have resolved the costliness of replacement of MPs. Lesotho's general election of May 2002 cost the country about an astronomical R70 million (11.2 million USD). Since the 2002 election the country has lost eight MPs due to death. Seven of these had been elected through the FPTP system and one through the PR system. The country has held about six by-elections already, each costing about R1 million (about USD 161 300). The seventh by-election was still to be organised at the time of writing.

Of the eight deceased MPs, three died due to accidents and the other five died of illness. This essentially means that the poverty-stricken mountain kingdom of Lesotho has spent about R7 million (USD 903 200) already, financing by-elections alone, just two years after the election of a parliament the tenure of which ends after five years.

4.3.3 COSTS ASSOCIATED WITH BY-ELECTIONS: SOUTH AFRICA

Compared with the countries that operate the FPTP electoral system, in South Africa the replacement of MPs does not impose financial costs or risk shifts in power in the legislatures because of its list PR system. The affected party simply reverts to its list of candidates and fills the vacancy. The seat cannot be contested by another party. The replacement of MPs in the South African legislature between 1994 and 2003 is illustrated in table 17. According to the data, 235 MPs were replaced due to resignation or death between 1994 and 2003. Of this total 182 MPs were replaced due to resignation and 23 due to death.

Table 17. Replacement of MPs in the South African legislature, 1994-2004

Year	Number of MPs	Replacement due to death	Affected parties
1994	12	2	ANC, NP, IFP
1995	15	1	ANC, NP, IFP
1996	32	1	ANC, NP, IFP
1997	31	2	ANC, NP, IFP, PAC, DP
1998	27	3	ANC, NNP, IFP
1999	45	2	ANC, NNP, IFP
2000	18	5	ANC, NNP, UDM, DP, IFP
2001	30	1	ANC, UDM, DP, IFP, FF, FA
2002	22	5	ANC, UDM, UCDP, IFP, NNP
2003	3	1	ANC
Total	**235**	**23**	...

Source: National Assembly, Republic of South Africa. Note that the size of South African Parliament is 400 MPs.

4.3.4 LOCAL GOVERNMENT BY-ELECTIONS IN SOUTH AFRICA

Local government by-elections in South Africa are governed by the 1998 Local Government Municipal Structures Act. The South African local government system comprises 312 metropolitan councils, 215 district councils and 1711 local councils. There are all in all about 3754 wards. Section 25 of the act stipulates conditions that call for a by-election as follows:

- If the IEC does not declare the result of the local government election within a period specified in the Electoral Act;
- If a court sets aside the election of a local government structure;
- If a council is dissolved; or
- If a vacancy in a ward occurs.

The electoral system used for local government elections and by-elections is as follows: (a) for local and municipal councils (styled Category A and Category B respectively) 50% of ward councillors are elected directly through the FPTP system and the other 50% through the PR model to achieve overall political proportionality; and (b) at the district level (styled Category C) 40% of the councillors are directly elected by eligible district residents, while 60% of the councillors are indirectly elected in that they are appointed representatives of local and municipal councils.

A majority of local government by-elections since 1999 have been due primarily to a vacancy at ward level caused by a number of factors, ranging from resignations, dismissal and floor-crossing to death of councillors.

The total cost of the 1994 general election in South Africa was R912 132 326 (about U$250 million) while the 1999 election cost is estimated at R529 210 483 (IEC, 1994; IEC, 1999). The total cost of the 2004 election had not been established by the time of writing.

In 2001 a total of 79 by-elections were held. Of these 27 were in KwaZulu-Natal and nine in Gauteng. In 2002 73 local government by-elections were organised and again top on the list was KwaZulu-Natal with 22 by-elections, followed by Northern Cape with nine. In 2003 the number of local government by-elections increased to 83, of which most were held in KwaZulu-Natal (21), followed by Northern Cape (nine), Western Cape (nine), Gauteng (eight) and Free State (eight). By May 2004 a total of 60 by-elections had been held. The causes for the by-elections range from resignations, floor-crossing and dismissals to death of councillors.

Due to the element of FPTP in its local-level elections, South Africa faces financial costs for by-elections, costs that are experienced on a national level in the other countries discussed previously. According to the IEC, each ward by-election costs about R30 000 (interview Hendrikse). Given this estimate, the total cost for by-elections in 2001 stood at R2.3 million. This figure declined slightly to about R2.2 million in 2002, but increased to about R2.5 million in 2003.

An analysis of the number of local-level by-elections in South Africa in the context of the HIV/AIDS epidemic runs into the same problems with data as mentioned above. The mere increase of deaths is, again, reason enough to explore this line of research further. The fact that KwaZulu-Natal, the province most affected by the epidemic (according to estimates by the Department of Health) also has the highest numbers of by-elections is obviously worth exploring in further depth. If the number of by-elections is found to be disproportional to its number of councillors it might indicate that the epidemic is one of the causes behind the death and resignation of so many local councillors. Whatever the cause, the KwaZulu-Natal electoral officer told us he was concerned about the high number of by-elections in the province, ie 70 by-elections over a period of three years (interview Mosery). See table 18.

Table 18. Number of by-elections for directly elected local councillors

Region	Size*	2001		2002		2003	
		actual	%	actual	%	actual	%
Eastern Cape	601	12	2.00	6	1.00	12	2.00
Free State	291	2	0.69	4	1.37	8	2.75
Gauteng	446	9	2.02	6	1.35	8	2.75
KwaZulu-Natal	748	27	3.61	22	2.94	21	2.81
Limpopo	402	2	2.24	5	1.75	4	1.50
Northern Cape	173	3	1.73	9	5.20	9	5.20
North West	327	7	2.14	8	2.45	6	1.83
Western Cape	340	8	2.35	6	1.76	9	2.65
Total	**3729**	**79**	**2.23**	**73**	**1.96**	**83**	**2.12**

Source: Electoral Commission. *Represents the % of the total number of counsellors who left during the year

4.4 ELECTORAL SYSTEM REFORM DEBATE IN SOUTH AFRICA SINCE 2002

Although electoral systems play such an important role in a democracy, countries hardly ever institutionalise regular reviews of their models and introduce reforms where necessary. Reynolds and Reilly advise appropriately that states should endeavour to review and deliberately design electoral systems that suit their own conditions with a view to deepening democratic governance. In doing so, they argue, it is advisable that eight key criteria are used to guide the process:

- Ensuring a representative parliament;
- Making elections accessible and meaningful;
- Providing incentives for conciliation;
- Facilitating stable and efficient government;
- Holding the government and representatives accountable;
- Encouraging "cross-cutting" political parties;
- Promoting a parliamentary opposition; and
- Cost and administrative capacity (2002:9-13).

For the purposes of this chapter one could also add a caveat that, while the above considerations are fairly adequate when countries consider electoral reform, it is equally important that countries undertake this delicate exercise bearing in mind the implications of such calamitous diseases such as HIV/AIDS. In other words, as countries reform their electoral models today they cannot ignore the impact of HIV/AIDS on the electoral model in place specifically and the governance realm in general.

The PR electoral model that South Africa has used since 1994 has, by all indications, served the country fairly well. First, it has certainly helped ensure broad representation of key political forces in the legislature. Second, and linked to the first point, the PR system has been a catalyst for increased gender balance or greater numbers of women participating in both parliament and the executive branch of government since 1994. Third, it has facilitated reconciliation and peace following a protracted violent conflict, thereby acting not only as a conflict management instrument, but also as a guarantor for political stability. Fourth, it has enhanced participation of the electorate in the political process, especially elections, by eliminating incidences of vote-wastage because all valid votes cast count towards the calculation of election results and parties thus earn their legislative seats in proportion to their electoral strength. Nevertheless, all these positive attributes of the PR model notwithstanding, there has been a lot of questioning of the PR model as currently applied in South Africa (see De Ville and Steytler, 1996), particularly since 1999 following the country's second democratic election (see Konrad Adenauer Foundation, 2003).

The general debate around the model prompted the government to appoint a task force on electoral reform primarily to advise on the best way forward for electoral system engineering in South Africa. Known as the Electoral Task Team (ETT), this commission was established on 20 March 2002 and headed by Dr Frederick van Zyl Slabbert. It had a fairly broad mandate: to (a) draft the new electoral legislation required by the Constitution and (b) formulate the parameters of new electoral legislation and draft it to prepare for the scheduled national and provincial elections of 2004 or any earlier election, should the need arise (Report of the Electoral Task Team, 2002:3). The terms of reference for the ETT were to:

- Identify the controlling constitutional parameters;
- Identify the salient and relevant aspects of the South African context;
- Identify the list of options available within the South African context;
- Canvass the preferences and views of relevant role-players and stakeholders with special regard to political parties in respect of the list of identified options;
- Develop specific proposals identifying the preferable electoral system to be canvassed with aforesaid role-players and stakeholders; and
- Formulate a draft bill for submission to Minister M Buthelezi (Report of the Electoral Task Team, 2002:4).

An international conference was organised jointly by the ETT, the Konrad-Adenauer-Stiftung and the Electoral Institute of Southern Africa (EISA) in Cape Town on 9-10 September 2002 to engage in this debate and bring on board regional and international perspectives and experiences. Even at the conference no consensus emerged regarding a preferred electoral model for South Africa because some participants agued for a MMP system, whereas others argued for the retention of the full List-PR system.

What is interesting, though, is that public opinion on the electoral reform was overwhelmingly in favour of the present List-PR system and its retention. A public opinion survey was undertaken by the Human Sciences Research Council (HSRC) of a total sample of 2 760 South African citizens of voting age selected randomly. According to Southall and Mattes (2002)

> *the survey asked … respondents a series of questions about their opinions of the current electoral system. Looking across the questions, it is clear that a substantial majority feels that, overall, the present system is fair. About three-quarters say they are "satisfied" with "the way we elect our government" (74%) and agree the system is "fair to all parties" (72%). Approximately two-thirds feel that "all voters were treated equally" in the 1999 elections (68%) and that "all parties were treated equally" in 1999 (63%).*

The Slabbert Commission conducted stakeholder workshops and interviewed political parties and other key stakeholders on the electoral system reform. The commission also engaged experts to undertake the survey on public opinion. However, that notwithstanding, in the end members of the task force were divided and two schools of thought informed the ultimate outcome.

A majority view emerged in favour of an MMP system which would introduce 69 multi-member constituencies from which 300 MPs would be elected via FPTP and 100 MPs would be elected on the basis of a closed-party list. A minority view emerged for the retention of the current system, arguing that its strengths outweigh its perceived weaknesses. As a result of the divergence of opinion within the commission, two reports emerged; the main report that advocated for the change of the model, and a minority report that called for the retention of the PR system.

The ETT submitted both reports to the minister of home affairs and the matter was subsequently presented to cabinet. According to Faure and Venter "the government's reaction to the ETT report was that the status quo would be maintained and that the newly elected government in 2004 would review the report and make a decision in preparation for the 2009 poll" (2003:8). All indications, therefore, point to a stark reality that one of the challenges that confront the ANC government following the 2004 election is the reform of the electoral model by revisiting the two reports that emerged from the Slabbert Commission. In fact electoral reform debate also will have to confront the new development introduced by the floor-crossing legislation in South Africa (see Southall, 2004).

There were various factors that influenced the government's decision not to undertake the electoral reforms of the majority position of the ETT. Roger Southall isolates five:

- The challenges posed by the introduction of a new model in respect of civic and voter education, especially as this was just in advance of the 2004 election;
- The perceived fairness and representativeness of the PR system, in particular its inherent virtues in a post-conflict South Africa;

- The system had become familiar and was considered simple to understand by the voters, compared with the proposed new MMP model;
- The system had proved itself conducive to gender equality in the political governance realm; and
- The very fact that the commission had not formed a solidified and unanimous opinion on the reform imperatives.

While the majority report emphasised the point that the PR is deficient in so far as accountability is concerned, hence the need for electoral system reform in South Africa, the point needs to be driven home that in fact accountability cannot be reduced to the workings of the electoral model alone as the larger political culture in South Africa also is key to its existence or absence. In other words, the problem of accountability in politics could as well be addressed and redressed by adopting measures that do not necessarily require the refinement of the electoral model. The main message carried by the minority report was simply that public opinion showed popular support for the PR system and political parties indicated preference for the retention of the model, hence there was no need to change the system. Furthermore, the minority report argued that the List-PR system in South Africa was good for the country because it was fair, inclusive and simple.

With the benefit of hindsight, the debate that was triggered by the ETT was quite frank and revealing in many respects and indeed considerably enriching for both policy and academic discourse on electoral models. However, the debate was severely lacking in terms of integrating the HIV/AIDS ramifications on the electoral system. Pretty much linked to the HIV/AIDS dimensions of elections and election outcomes and replacement of MPs, the debate lacked much in-depth analysis on the costs of elections, especially by-elections. On this score, it is therefore worth reiterating the following realities of the HIV/AIDS epidemic in respect of elections and electoral engineering:

- Much as the FPTP electoral model is reputed for accountability, it tends to be fairly costly financially, administratively and politically, especially when it comes to the replacement of MPs through by-elections;
- While the PR system is reputed for broadening representation, it is less costly financially and administratively (although still costly politically) when it comes to the replacement of MPs through party lists; and
- If the experience of Lesotho that has just adopted the MMPR electoral model is anything to go by, this system does not adequately address the financial, administrative and political cost of replacing MPs.

The conclusion that can be drawn from these broad observations is that as the HIV/AIDS epidemic takes its toll the political elite is bound to be affected too. Thus, the question to ponder is how South Africa engineers its electoral machinery in such a way as to ensure minimal impact of the pandemic on elected representatives in the National Assembly. It would thus be useful if, when the electoral system reform debate resumes once again, that various critical issues, including HIV/AIDS, are taken on board. If our judgement that the replacement of MPs is one of the critical challenges for the democracy project in the era of HIV/AIDS holds water then it is only fair to argue that South Africa is likely to be better served by retaining its current PR system, while institutionalising accountability mechanisms by focusing on re-ordering the political culture.

However, it also is possible that the electoral reform process will not be revisited, even now that the 2004 election is over, for as Paul Graham rightly puts it:

> *... there is no commitment from the political leadership for such a reform process. This can be triggered only if Parliament so desires. However, the last thing that we can expect from MPs is to have the nerve to question and critique the system that earned them parliamentary seats. Let us recall that British Prime Minister Tony Blair promised to prioritise the issue of electoral reforms when he assumed power. It is now eight years and the Blair government has never tabled the issue before parliament (interview, Graham).*

It would thus come as no surprise if no further efforts are made by the South African government towards reform measures.

CONCLUSION

This chapter has discussed the possible linkages between the electoral system and the HIV/AIDS epidemic in South Africa, highlighting comparative insights from the SADC region. The chapter introduced the discussion with general remarks on elections and electoral systems. The significance of elections and electoral systems to a vibrant and robust democratic governance was emphasised. We observed that while elections denote the process of choosing national leaders to run the affairs of a particular nation on behalf of the electorate, an electoral system simply refers to the method of choosing the leaders and translating votes cast into parliamentary seats.

In both cases it has been noted that the HIV/AIDS epidemic does have its own impact and this impact in turn affects the institutionalisation of democratic governance. After introducing the two major electoral systems that are dominant in the SADC region, namely the FPTP system and the PR (List-PR and MMP) systems, we have established that an argument could be made that on average the countries that operate the FPTP system are hardest hid by the adverse effects of HIV/AIDS relative to those operating the PR (especially those operating the List-PR) system.

The South African electoral system was put under the spotlight and in this regard our assessment is that whereas at the national and provincial levels the List-PR system might have stood the country in good stead in respect of the impact of HIV/AIDS in many respects, its local government system has not spared it from the ravages of the epidemic by and large. Put another way, compared with the FPTP electoral system which is prevalent in a majority of the SADC states, the PR model that South Africa has used since 1994 stands the country in good stead when it comes to the replacement of MPs given that the system does not require by-elections and as such it tends to be less costly. However, while this situation exists at the national and provincial legislatures level, it is not necessarily so at local government level where the country operates a hybrid system combining elements of PR and FPTP systems. It is imperative that as South Africa considers electoral engineering aimed at reforming its electoral system following the 2004 election, issues around the impact of HIV/AIDS on governance should also be seriously considered.

Four major conclusions of the chapter emanating from the observations above are therefore in order. First, the replacement of MPs translates into enormous financial cost for countries operating the FPTP and MMP systems due to the requirement for holding by-elections and this affects South Africa in respect of local government by-elections.

Second, the replacement of MPs does amount to a political cost (which might not be quantifiable) to affected political parties irrespective of the electoral system in use and South Africa is no exception to this general rule.

Third, the replacement of MPs might distort the configuration of power in parliament and this is mainly the case with countries operating the FPTP system. This does not apply to South Africa. Fourth, and finally, by-elections might (and often do) have a tendency to reduce the degree of political mandate given to MPs to run affairs of the nation on behalf of the electorate in that, compared with general and local government elections, by-elections are generally marked by lower voter turnout.

An increase in the number of deceased and sick persons will have an impact on the core functions of the IEC. The delimitation of voting districts and the registration of voters will be affected as deceased persons must be taken off the voters' roll, which also affects the delimitation of voting districts as well as the arrangements for sick persons that we currently have in place (interview, Hendrickse).

Chapter 5

Electoral Administration and Management in South Africa

Democratic elections are generally managed by a specialised administrative structure within the public service since the overall integrity of the electoral process should be guaranteed by the state beyond the reach of any partisan interests. Any weaknesses in the electoral process could be interpreted as an indicator of a lack of commitment to democracy itself by the state and/or the incumbent government (Olaleye, 2003), but deficiencies also of course can have other causes. In the context of HIV/AIDS it is, therefore, important to develop an understanding of the nature and extent of the challenges posed by the epidemic to the effective administration of elections by such electoral commissions.

A lack of understanding in this regard will lead to insufficient interventions that might undermine the effective administration of free and fair elections. Such a problematic development would, in turn, threaten the legitimacy of the electoral process as such and by implication undermine all efforts to develop a sustainable democracy.

In this chapter we shall explore how the HIV/AIDS epidemic might impact on the effective fulfilment of the mandate given to the South African Independent Electoral Commission (IEC). Has the IEC already started to experience some effects of the epidemic? Is it aware of and prepared for how such effects might increase in the next few years as the epidemic moves into a phase when its consequences will be increasingly felt in terms of AIDS-related illness and mortality? Is the IEC prepared in ways that would apply to any and all workplaces and has it developed a strategic plan to avoid having its core function undermined by the epidemic in future national elections?

We shall attempt to address these and related questions by firstly describing the legislative and institutional framework for the IEC's administration and regulation of elections in South Africa. On the basis of the findings and hypotheses presented in existing research we shall then investigate how the IEC might be directly affected by the epidemic and what the commission is seeking to do to effectively counter such negative effects.

5.1 STRUCTURES, STAFF AND LEGAL FRAMEWORK OF THE IEC

In the transition from apartheid to democracy it was recognised by the negotiating parties that there would be a need to set up an independent body to manage the elections to ensure that they would be free and fair (Asmal and De Ville, 1994). Two authorities were created accordingly – the IEC and an independent authority to regulate broadcasting, the Independent Communication Authority of South Africa (Icasa) – which had their independence enshrined in the Constitution.[12] The IEC was first established by statute (the Independent Electoral Commission Act, No 150 of 1993) as an interim body with the mandate to organise and rule on the "free-ness and fairness" of the first democratic elections in

April 1994. It was subsequently made a permanent body through the promulgation of the Electoral Commission Act, No 51 of 1996 with the mission to strengthen, promote and safeguard constitutional democracy through the delivery of free and fair elections in which every voter is able to record his or her informed choices (IEC 2004a).

5.1.1 STRUCTURES AND STAFF

With its head office in Pretoria and provincial offices in each of the nine provinces, the IEC has a multi-level structure, which is headed by five commissioners who have been appointed in terms of para 6 of the Electoral Act. The current commissioners are Dr Bam, Professor Vilikazi, Judge Hussain, Ms Mpumlwana and Mr van der Merwe (IEC 2004d). The act further provides that the commission is to be headed by a chief electoral officer, a position currently filled by Advocate Pansy Tlakula, who is assisted by a deputy. Each of the nine provincial offices is headed by a provincial electoral officer. In June 2004 the IEC had altogether 116 full-time staff at the national office and seven to 13 staff at each of the nine provincial offices (a total of 92 provincial staff).[13] Each of the nine provincial offices works in association with local government Municipal Electoral Officers (MEOs). It appears that MEOs are employed by local governments but work under the direction of the provincial IEC office – although this was not completely clear.[14] For example, in KwaZulu-Natal there are 51 municipal offices and 102 MEOs (interview Mosery). Finally, temporary staff assist the IEC during periods of national and provincial elections. During the 2004 elections an additional 224 staff were added to the permanent staff and 215 460 electoral officials were appointed in terms of section 74 of the Electoral Act to assist with the management of voting (IEC June 2004). In terms of recruiting temporary staff to assist with elections the IEC has a formal arrangement with the Department of Education so that 98% of the presiding officers and deputy presiding officers are drawn from the ranks of teachers (interview Mosery). The temporary staff employed during national and provincial elections is divided by the IEC into three categories (interview Mosery):

Casuals are people who are employed to work in the voting station on election days. They are generally teachers employed at the school being used as a polling station;

Presiding officers and *deputy presiding officers* are responsible for managing each voting station. They are also generally teachers; and

Area supervisors are generally municipal staff who manage a number of voting districts.

The multi-level structure of the IEC is clarified further in figure 3 on the next page.

Figure 3. The multi-level structure of the IEC

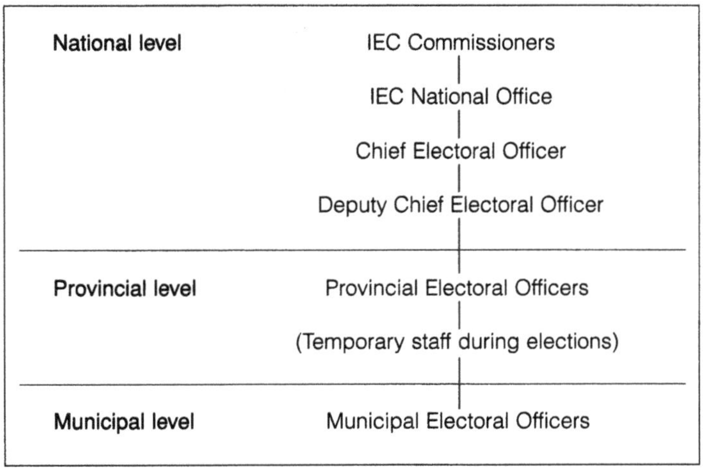

5.1.2 LEGISLATIVE FRAMEWORK

The legal framework for managing elections in South Africa is set out in an extensive array of legislation. As mentioned above the commission was enshrined in the Constitution to ensure that elections would be managed by an independent body. It is thus one of the six state institutions that are identified and protected in chapter nine of the Constitution, all of which are mandated to support our constitutional democracy.[15] All these bodies are subject only to the Constitution and the law and they must be impartial and exercise their powers and perform their functions without fear, favour or prejudice (section 181[2]). All other organs of the state and government departments are, according to section 181(3), obliged to "assist and protect" the "Chapter Nine" institutions, but without seeking to intrude on their autonomy.

The IEC's three core functions, set out in section 190(1) of the Constitution, are:

- To "manage elections of national, provincial and municipal legislative bodies in accordance with national legislation;
- Ensure that theses elections are free and fair; and
- Declare the results of those elections within a period that must be prescribed by national legislation and which is as short as is reasonably possible."

These core functions must be seen in the light of the constitutional rights to vote in free and fair elections (section 19). In other words the IEC is the mechanism which has been created to ensure that the right to vote can be exercised. Some writers argue that the primary obligations imposed by sections 19(2) and (3)[16] of the Constitution are positive ones requiring the state (through its IEC) to take steps to ensure that the right of every adult citizen to vote is fulfilled (De Waal, 2003). The Constitutional Court has confirmed this interpretation of the Constitution (through its decisions in *New National Party of South Africa v Government of the Republic of South Africa*, para 118 and *August and Another v*

Electoral Commission, para 16). This means that when the IEC makes policy decisions regarding matters, such as where to place voting stations, setting the hours for voting and describing the requirements for proof of identity, the legislature and the IEC should seek to enhance democracy and not limit it (*New National Party case*, para 122). This positive obligation on the IEC to ensure that every citizen's right to vote is fulfilled will be discussed in more detail later on in this chapter since it has implications for the IEC in the context of the HIV/AIDS epidemic.

The constitutional provisions relating to the electoral commission are described in more detail in the Electoral Commission Act (No 51 of 1996) which makes provision for the establishment of the Electoral Commission to "manage elections for national, provincial and local legislative bodies and referenda". The act states that the commission is an independent body, which is subject only to the Constitution and the law (section 3[1]). Its objectives are to "strengthen constitutional democracy and promote democratic electoral processes" (section 4). The powers, duties and functions of the commission are set out in section 5 of the act and include, among others, to:

- "Manage any election [...];
- Ensure that any election is free and fair;
- Promote conditions conducive to free and fair elections [...];
- Compile and maintain voters' rolls by means of a system of registering of eligible voters by utilizing data available from government sources [...];
- Undertake and promote research into electoral matters [...];
- Continually review electoral legislation and proposed electoral legislation, to make recommendations in connection therewith [...];
- Appoint appropriate public administration in any sphere of government to conduct elections when necessary."

These functions clearly show that the IEC has a complex dual role; that of being both a manager and a regulator of elections. The way in which the IEC should undertake these core functions is set out in the Electoral Act, No 73 of 1998 and the Electoral Laws Amendment Act, No 34 of 2003. These acts should be read with the Local Government Municipal Electoral Act, No 27 of 2000 which regulates local government elections. The core functions of the IEC that are defined by these acts include:

- Maintaining a voters' roll. Section 5 of the Electoral Act states that there is an obligation on the chief electoral officer to compile and maintain a national common voters' roll. Sections 5 and 6 of the Local Government Municipal Electoral Act states that the national common voters' roll will be used during local government elections. However for the purposes of such elections the chief electoral officer must ensure that it is broken into segments for each municipality;
- Organising voter registration. Section 6(1) of the Electoral Act provides that to register as a voter a person must be a South African citizen and have an identity document. Furthermore to vote every citizen must register in the prescribed manner in the voting district in which s/he is ordinarily resident (section 7[1]). The IEC describes the place where a voter is ordinarily resident as being the place where s/he lives and to where s/he returns after temporary

absences (IEC, 2004c) If a voter leaves the place where he or she is ordinarily resident then s/he must apply to the IEC to change his/her voter registration details (section 9[1]).

- Organising voting. The Electoral Act provides in section 36(1) that the IEC must prescribe the voting hours on election day. The chief electoral officer is duty bound to ensure that these are publicised in the media (section 36[3]). Section 60(1) of the Electoral Act requires the commission to establish voting districts in which the polling will take place. The act also prescribes the criteria that should be used when making these determinations (section 61). The criteria mentioned include: the number and distribution of eligible voters, the accessibility of voting stations, the availability of transport and geographic or physical features that might impede access to voting. Within each voting district the IEC is obliged to establish voting stations. Section 64(2) refers to the factors that should be taken into account in deciding where to place such voting stations and they include an assessment of the "general facilities at these venues". There is no specific mention of the need to ensure that there are facilities for disabled or sick people. There are two relevant provisions in the Electoral Act which relate to assisting disabled persons to vote. Firstly, a registered voter might apply for a special vote if s/he is unable to vote at a voting station within the district where s/he is registered due to physical infirmity, disability or pregnancy (section 33[1]). And secondly, "a person" may assist a voter who requires help at the voting station due to a physical disability (section 39[2]) with the process of voting, provided that the voter has a physical disability, has asked for assistance and his/her helper is over the age of 18. The Local Government Municipal Electoral Act states that unless the IEC determines otherwise the voting hours will be from 7.30 am until 21.00 (section 45). Section 48 provides that assistance must be given to certain voters. In this regard another person might assist a voter who is physically disabled or who has requested assistance. On a local level the law makes no provision for special votes.
- Observing the elections. Section 84(3) of the Electoral Act provides that certain people might be accredited by the IEC as observers of the election. Likewise, section 41 of the Local Government Municipal Electoral Act states that people might apply to be observers of a local government election.

5.2 THE INTERNAL IMPACT OF HIV/AIDS

5.2.1 REVIEW OF THE LITERATURE

This section will first review some literature and discuss the way in which the epidemic is hypothesised to affect the staff within electoral institutions, referred to as the internal impact of HIV/AIDS. The way in which the services provided by electoral institutions might be affected by the epidemic, the external impact of HIV/AIDS, will be discussed under section 5.3. Since there is no literature that specifically addresses the internal impact on electoral commissions, we shall refer to literature that discusses possible effects on state bureaucracies more broadly, some of which might be less relevant to the IEC. The following section seeks to apply the more generally formulated impacts in the literature to the specific circumstances of the IEC to provide a basis for an informed discussion of how the epidemic risk will negatively affect the commission over the next few years.

The literature identifies a number of ways that the epidemic is likely to have an impact on the internal functioning of workplaces such as state bureaucracies. It is important to point out, however, that since most of these discussions assume that HIV-positive employees do not have access to effective and comprehensive treatment, the scenarios we sketch out in this section will obviously become less problematic should such treatment become available for the vast majority of infected employees in the near future.

INCREASED LEVELS OF MORBIDITY

As infected employees become ill they will take additional sick leave, which will disrupt operational activities. For example, the human resources department at eTekwini Municipality reported that in its Parks, Recreation and Culture Department they had a 32% turnover of staff over a period of six months (Manning, 2003), which has implications for both productivity and costs. The effects of such disruptions will be amplified when more qualified and experienced employees are absent since they are more difficult to replace on a temporary basis (Whiteside, 2000). The Public Service is likely to be seriously affected by these developments. In a report commissioned by the Department of Public Service and Administration, entitled the *Impact and Action Report* (2000), it was projected that by 2011 a full 27% of skilled civil servants in South Africa will be infected with HIV, see table 19.

Table 19. Projected percentage of HIV infection levels by grade

	1997	2005	2011
Low skilled	3	14	17
Skilled	4	20	27
Highly skilled	2	15	22
Supervisory	2	7	11
Managers	2	7	12
Senior managers	1	7	10

Source: DPSA 2000.

Table 20 shows the possible impact on morbidity if no measures are introduced to mitigate the impact of HIV. With regard to electoral commissions it has been noted that as they require a pool of skilled people if elections are to be effectively managed, the loss of such personnel, particularly highly skilled staff, poses a direct threat to

Table 20. Projected percentage annual AIDS deaths within government departments[17]

	1997	2005	2011
Water/Forestry	1	1.5	2.7
Govt Admin	1	1.5	2.6
National Govt	1	1.4	2.4
Justice	1	1.4	2.5
Home Affairs	1	1.4	2.4
Foreign Affairs	1	0.9	1.7
Labour	1	1.3	2.6

Source: DPSA 2000.

the competence of commissions.

Actual increases in AIDS-related illnesses that approximate these estimates will inevitably lead to corresponding increases in costs for employment benefits such as medical schemes (George, 2003).

MORTALITY OR EARLY RETIREMENT

The *Impact and Action Report* also projected that AIDS will have become the leading cause of death among civil servants by the end of 2002, resulting in 250 000 deaths by 2012 or 23% of the current 1.1 million strong workforce. Table 21 shows the projected annual AIDS deaths in the public service as detailed in the *Impact and Action Report.*

Table 21. Non-intervention scenario projections based on the Metropolitan Doyle model

	2001	2005	2010
Percentage of SA workforce (16-59) HIV+	18.02	22.35	24.08
Percentage of SA workforce AIDS sick	0.93	1.98	2.91
New AIDS cases p.a.	235 000	397 000	541 000
Life expectancy: females	52	43	37
Life expectancy: males	49	43	38

Source: George, 2003.

A sector that has been identified as being particularly at risk of infection with HIV is teachers. A recent study undertaken in KwaZulu-Natal estimated an increase in AIDS-related deaths among educators from 0.64% in 1999 to around 5% by 2010 (Badcock-Walters, Desmond, Wilson & Heard, 2003). This is of significance to the IEC since it relies particularly on the assistance of teachers on election day; high rates of infection leading to higher than average rates of mortality is a potential threat to the effective administration of elections due to an increased loss of the particular skills and experiences earned by those who have worked for the IEC in previous elections (Mattes 2003; Chirambo and Caesar, 2003). The loss of such employees requires an appropriate replacement to be selected and trained, which implies an extra cost to the organisation. For highly qualified staff this is often difficult, particularly in developing economies with skills shortages. One author predicts that this will sharply increase the remuneration budgets of organisations and state departments (Smart, 1999).

An additional impact that is impossible to quantify is the process of mentoring and skills transfer which must take place when new staff are brought into the organisation (Barrett Grant, Strode and Smart, 2002). Manning illustrates this by reporting on an interview with the Durban Fire Department where it noted that although it only takes three months to train replacement fire officers, it takes years to develop fire fighters to the point where they are experienced enough to pass on key skills and knowledge to younger staff members through informal training and mentoring (2003). Adding to this problem is the fact that staff who are ill leave their jobs and might die with little warning because of the stigma that

HIV carries and the discrimination they fear being subjected to, thus preventing a smooth transition of skills transfer from taking place. Mattes warns us what these problems might imply for election authorities such as the IEC in southern Africa:

> *The loss of non-partisan supervisory officials, combined with the complicated voter registration procedures of southern Africa's multiparty systems, will increase opportunities for voter fraud (2003).*

INCREASED ABSENTEEISM

As the HIV/AIDS epidemic advances, increases in AIDS-related illnesses and deaths will lead to increased absenteeism as employees are too sick to come to work or they attend funerals for family members, friends and colleagues or take time off to care for sick family members (Whiteside, 2000).

LOWER STAFF MORALE

A fear of infection and death might lead to increased suspicion of others, as well as resistance to shouldering the additional responsibilities for colleagues who are off sick, away from work or newly recruited and not yet fully functional.

In the eTekwini Municipality case study it was noted that human resource staff were burdened with the emotional impact of dealing with many young staff members dying and leaving behind children and families (Manning, 2003).

EMPLOYMENT EQUITY PROFILE

Considering that those most affected by HIV are black women it is probable that the negative impacts of the epidemic on the workplace also will affect the employment equity profile of organisations negatively, but very little has been written yet on this point.

5.2.2 INTERNAL IMPACT OF HIV/AIDS ON THE IEC

Every workplace needs to respond to the impact HIV/AIDS will have on their employees and on the services they provide. Our review of the literature above gives some more precise indications of what the nature of the impact might be. In this section we shall see how these general impacts translate to the workplace that is the IEC by investigating its staff profile and turnover.

Generally it is of course the case that all workplaces are only as vulnerable to the effects of HIV/AIDS as the degree to which their individual employees engage in behaviours, sexual or not, that put them at risk for infection. It is nevertheless possible to argue that some workplaces are more vulnerable than others due to the extent that their staff profile overlaps with the groups in the population that we know have a higher rate of infection than others. This is the case for the IEC in terms of the following three points:

- A slight majority of its staff is female, the gender most affected by the epidemic;
- The age structure of its staff shows that 85% fall into the age group that is most vulnerable to HIV infection (see further below);
- Almost all temporary staff are teachers, a profession known to be hit hard by the epidemic.

With the following age structure of its permanent staff – four staff 18-24 years; 178 staff 25-49 years; 28 staff 50-60 years – the IEC is vulnerable to the much higher HIV prevalence and effects of AIDS among young and middle-aged adults. This vulnerability is aggravated by the fact that most temporary staff are likely to fall within the same age brackets, which is likely to reduce the IEC's ability to rely on the same temporary staff to bring experiences and skills from their work with administrating previous elections into the administration of future elections.

In the past three years a total of four permanent staff died while employed by the IEC. Three of these deaths occurred in 2003, a figure that translates to roughly 1.44% of its permanent staff that year. Although at a very low level in terms of numbers of actual deaths, it should be noted that the figure corresponds with the estimated number of deaths for government departments as detailed in table 21 above. In making this observation we need to make it absolutely clear that we do not in any way wish to imply that any of the three permanent staff at the IEC who died during 2003 died from AIDS. Our point here is merely to highlight a correspondence between estimates of the impact of AIDS and actual occurrences on a more general level (see table 22).

Table 22. IEC staff turnover

Year	Number of staff leaving the IEC	Death*	Resignation	Other unknown
2001	153	1	3	149
2002	10	0	10	0
2003	15	3	12	0
Total	178	4	25	149

Source: IEC, 2004.
*This represents the percentage of staff who died whilst still in service.

The data made available to us from the IEC provides us with no real basis from which to comment conclusively on what impact AIDS might have had on its internal structures in terms of loss of staff. If anything the impact seems to have been relatively minor. This conclusion is, however, not very solid as the following information would be needed to reach more definite conclusions:

- Temporary staff. We were unable to establish the impact of HIV on the temporary election staff employed by the IEC. The commission uses a system called the Electoral Staff System that captures the details of all temporary election officers to allow the IEC to approach the same individuals to assist with each new election. The system does not, however, keep records of how many of these individuals were not available for subsequent elections (interview Hendrickse).

- Specialist staff. It is not clear how many of the staff who left or died in the past few years were specialists in any of the key sections of the IEC – information technology, electoral logistics, voters' roll management and electoral training – and what their departure implied for the effective functioning of those key sections.
- Staff absenteeism. No information was obtained in terms of numbers or trends in staff absenteeism.

More comprehensive research into the internal effects of the epidemic on the functioning of the IEC will have to take into account this additional information to the extent it is at all possible to attain.

5.2.3 The IEC's response to the internal impact

The IEC has started to respond to the impact of HIV/AIDS on its internal functions. It developed and adopted an HIV/AIDS policy in May 2002 and a review of the policy is planned for 2004. The commission is also busy developing a skills succession plan to deal with the possible loss of highly skilled employees (interview Hendrickse). The policy development was gone through a consultative process with the provincial offices although staff did not actively participate in the process more generally. Mr Mawetu Mosery, provincial electoral officer in KwaZulu-Natal commented on this process:

> *Most staff did not see it as relevant to them as they did not believe that they are at risk for infection with HIV. Resultantly there has been very little buy in from staff (interview Mosery).*

The IEC's stated vision in the policy is to mobilise its staff to engage actively in:

- Prevention programmes;
- Counselling and supporting infected and affected colleagues and their families and where possible supporting the provision of education on issues related to the epidemic;
- Providing resources and leadership to implement HIV/AIDS and associated wellness programmes for the workplace;
- The creation of a non-discriminatory environment that will break down stigma to ensure that the epidemic can be addressed and support provided in a sensitive and humane manner within the working environment; and
- The protection of confidentiality within the workplace for members whose HIV status is known.

While these policy ambitions are constructive there are some shortcomings that need to be highlighted. As the policy applies only to permanent staff, it does not address the needs or place an obligation on temporary staff or the MEOs. In developing the policy it was assumed that all local governments have their own HIV/AIDS policies that would cover the MEOs (interview Mosery). Currently there are therefore no programmes or policies in place to manage the possible impact of HIV on these categories of staff. Secondly, costs are not addressed in the policy at all. Thirdly, the policy does not explicitly ensure staff the right to ARV treatment. However, with the roll-out of the Department of Health's National Treatment Plan and the availability of ARVs through medical aid schemes all staff should be able to access treatment on an individual basis through either the private or public sector.

Over and above its policy statement the IEC also has limited HIV/AIDS programmes in place that are co-ordinated by an HIV/AIDS focal point person in each office. The more common interventions of this kind are to ensure that condoms are available in the bathrooms and that HIV/AIDS information is available in all offices. It was, however, noted by Mosery that these interventions were not particularly prioritised; they gained attention with some additional activities around World AIDS Day. Two areas in which the IEC has done little or no work relate to promoting voluntary testing and counselling, as well as creating an environment that reduces stigma (interview Mosery).

5.3 THE EXTERNAL IMPACT OF HIV/AIDS

The literature identifies a number of different ways in which the HIV epidemic could impact on electoral commissions' core functions. In particular the literature shows that service delivery within any organisation might be negatively affected – not only due to the number of infected employees who are unable to work at their full capacity, but also due to the increased demand for certain services. In this regard services in remote areas and disadvantaged communities might be particularly vulnerable to absenteeism or deaths among staff because of shortages of skilled staff and resource constraints (Barrett Grant, Strode and Smart, 2002). Furthermore, planning for future service demands is complicated by the rapidly changing demographics of HIV/AIDS and uncertainty about how it will impact on service needs. We shall discuss the implications of this under two headings: the pre-election phase and the polling phase.

5.3.1 PRE-ELECTION PHASE

Commentators have noted that sharp increases in mortality due to AIDS will pose significant problems for the correct and timely compilation and maintenance of the voters' roll. Where the electoral commission does not manage this as well as it should, the inaccuracies on the voters' roll open the door for electoral fraud. For example, it has been estimated by the Malawian Electoral Commission that roughly 100 000 (or 2%) of the total number of voters on its roll are deceased.

Where the process by which births and deaths are not efficiently and correctly recorded electronically in a central population register but where each voter's status must be verified by a district commissioner, village headman, chief or another prominent person, the process is bound to consume much resources and time without necessarily ending up being correct (Ngwembe 2003). Most commentators hold the view that the problems in Malawi are replicated to some degree in most if not all of the countries in southern Africa. The problem is however not necessarily easily fixed through reforms within the electoral commission alone, but arguably requires an effective and efficient public service more generally (Olaleye 2003).

The literature also discusses ways in which the epidemic might impact on voter registration. People with AIDS (or any other serious decease) who are bedridden will have serious difficulties with registering for elections if this implies travel of any kind. Registering might also become difficult for AIDS orphans since they often lack proper birth certificates which they need to get the necessary identification documents for registration on the voters' roll. Furthermore, since many impoverished families are strained even further by the effects of the epidemic they might be unable to afford the costs associated with travelling to town to obtain an identity document and to register as a voter. Registration rates also might go down due to voter apathy as a result of the epidemic, which appears to have been the case in the most recent Zambian election (Chirambo 2003: Mattes 2003; Chirambo and Caesar 2003). The effect on registration of these factors becomes even more problematic where the law or a shortage of resources does not allow officers of electoral commissions to register people through home visits. If, in addition, people who move to another part of the country – often those suffering from AIDS-related illnesses move to get home-based care from those in the extended family living in the family's rural base – have to reregister to cast their votes in their new location.

5.3.2 POLLING PHASE

When the actual elections are under way during the polling phase those who never managed to register for reasons related to AIDS are of course lost to the electoral process. But registered voters also might end up not making use of their right to vote by choice or circumstance due to one or more of the following factors. Firstly, only if the voting stations are open for long hours during one or more days will those who have difficulties with transport have a real chance to get there in time, a problem that often is more acute in rural areas. Secondly, special provisions have to be made to ensure that those voters who have special needs due to pregnancy, or any illness or disability can cast their votes without having to wait in long queues and, when necessary, cast their votes with the assistance of an electoral officer or trusted friend. A third and final problem that might hinder participation for reasons that are directly linked to AIDS has to do with the need for voters to enter a public space, ie the actual voting station, to cast their votes.

While in most cases this is not a problem – as long as some voters get assistance to reach that space and to move within it – the problem with the stigma attached to the epidemic presents a unique and very problematic set of obstacles that are likely to hinder participation from registered voters who suffer from AIDS-related illnesses.

We shall return to this issue below in chapter ten where we listen directly to some of the stories and experiences of such voters as they sought to cast their votes in the most recent South African election. Suffice it to say here that electoral commissions must consider how to convince voters suffering from AIDS-related illnesses that staff at the voting stations will do their best to counter any prejudice and maltreatment that might be directed at them while at the voting station. Let us now move from this more general discussion to looking at the specific conditions in South Africa.

5.3.3 EXTERNAL IMPACT ON THE IEC

There is a clear understanding in South Africa among the relevant authorities of the importance of an accurate voter's roll in protecting the legitimacy of elections – the point was made recently in a Constitutional Court judgment (Minister of Home Affairs v NICRO and Others, at para 71). The IEC is obviously central to the process by which such accuracy is ensured. Before any election in South Africa, be it national, provincial or local, the IEC has to certify the voters' roll. In this verification process the IEC establishes if there have been any changes to the status of any registered voters in terms of death, migration or citizenship. Everyone on the voters' roll who is marked as deceased on the National Population Register, which is managed by the Department of Home Affairs, is identified as being invalid on the voters' roll and is electronically removed by the system (interview Mzaidume). The human side of this job was highlighted in a letter to the Natal Witness, which noted with sadness that in the task of "tidying up" the voters' roll the authors had observed that most people who were being removed were between the ages of 18 and 30. (See appendix A for the full text of the letter.) Chapter nine will explore in some depth the mortality profiles of all the registered voters who were removed from the voters' roll between 1999 and 2003.

All indications are that the registration process in South Africa for the 2004 elections went relatively smoothly; all major political parties expressed satisfaction with the outcome of the registration process (The Star, 26 January 2004). Our inquiries to senior officials in the IEC suggested that the IEC had not experienced any of the possible impacts in the pre-election phase that we discussed above to a noticeable degree. The IEC established 17 000 registration points staffed by 50 271 staff throughout South Africa to make voter registration accessible. Furthermore MEOs were given the responsibility of ensuring that people who were in hospital or bed-ridden were visited at home to facilitate their registration as voters (IEC, 2004b). The IEC recommended that to further facilitate registration, voters should be able to register electronically. Political parties, however, opposed this, arguing that it would increase the possibility of voter fraud (interview, Mosery).

IEC planning for the polling phase also suggests that substantial resources were committed to ensure that none of the problems discussed above undermined the legitimacy of the election. The IEC had planned for voting to take place during long hours on polling day at 16 966 voting stations throughout the country. Voting stations were generally quite accessible. The average distance between the outer-boundary of a voting district and voting stations was 7.5 – 8 km in urban areas and 12.5 – 13km in rural areas. And, finally, voters with special needs were able to cast their votes a day ahead of election day, thus avoiding having to queue for long hours. Michael Hendrickse, senior manager in the Electoral Democracy, Training and Legal Services Division of the IEC, elaborated on other measures that had been taken to help people with special needs to cast their votes:

> *As a rule, disabled and sick persons are given preference and moved to the front of the queue, if there is one. A person with a physical disability may be assisted to cast their ballot inside the voting station by another person at the request of that voter. Braille ballot papers are made available at each voting station to allow a blind person to vote without assistance if he or she so wishes. Accessibility of the voting station by a person in a wheelchair is highlighted when deciding on a venue and each voting station has at least one voting compartment/booth that is accessible to a person in a wheelchair (interview Hendrickse).*

The IEC further ensures that water is available at every voting station and has encouraged the Department of Health also to deploy staff at polling stations to help those with special medical needs. So far the IEC has had little success with this suggestion as the department argues it would prevent its staff from voting since medical personnel cannot vote on a separate day, such as some military and police personnel in terms of the Electoral Act (interview, Mosery). To round off this section it is important to note that our brief comments here on how the IEC managed the pre-election and polling phases are not based on a comprehensive and independent evaluation by us, but rather on our own more general observations and on the information provided by the IEC itself. A more thorough analysis will have to be the focus of another research report.

5.3.4 THE SPECIAL VOTE

The most constructive institutional device that the IEC had to counter the potential effects of the epidemic was the "special vote". The Electoral Act (33[1]) (a) provides for the IEC to make arrangements for the physically disabled, infirm or pregnant; those absent from South Africa on government service; election staff; and those absent from the country on holiday, business or tertiary education to cast special votes. Applications had to be lodged by 8 April 2004.

Special voters were enabled to cast their ballots between 9am and 5pm on 12 and 13 April 2004, before the rest of the country went to the polls on April 14. A total of 651 438 special votes were cast during the 2004 general election. Table 23 shows the provincial breakdown of special votes.

Table 23. Special votes cast in 2004

	Total number of special votes	Special votes / registered (%)	Special votes / actual votes (%)
Western Cape	26 976	1.2	1.7
Eastern Cape	103 046	3.6	4.5
Northern Cape	15 544	3.6	4.7
Free State	49 526	3.7	4.8
KwaZulu-Natal	59 471	1.6	2.1
North West	103 302	5.9	7.6
Gauteng	130 835	2.8	3.7
Mpumalanga	76 293	5.3	6.6
Limpopo	80 278	3.7	4.6
National	651 438	3.2	4.1

Source: Independent Electoral Commission

The IEC has not compiled information on the reasons that applicants gave for requesting the special vote (interview Mosery). We are therefore not in a position to say with any precision or on the basis of independent analysis whether the delivery of special votes matched the expressed demand, or whether any applicants gave AIDS as the reason for their requests. As we shall show below, however, there are no strong indications that the special vote was used to a larger degree in the provinces with higher estimates of HIV infection or projections of AIDS-related illnesses. The main problems the IEC encountered with special votes were the high cost of facilitating such votes and that the system was abused by people who did not really qualify for a special vote. There also were security problems relating to maintaining the secrecy of the ballot and ensuring that no pressure was placed on voters. Political parties frequently disputed special votes because of these concerns (interview Mosery).

The "special vote" is a useful institutional arrangement to ensure, as far as possible, that people are not disenfranchised by being ill, disabled or pregnant. The mere fact that it exists and was delivered to more than 650 000 voters in the last election is a powerful indication of the commitment by the South African authorities to making democratic participation through the vote as inclusive as possible. In the context of our investigation here, however, it seems as if the IEC was a little too quick to refer to the special vote when asked about its response to the HIV/AIDS epidemic. As we shall see in chapters below, other information indicates that more needs to be done before the IEC can be said to have formulated a comprehensive response to the epidemic. There is no lack of insight into the magnitude and nature of the problem facing the IEC among its senior staff. Hendrickse argued that:

> *An increase in the number of deceased and sick persons will have an impact on the core functions of the IEC. The delimitation of voting districts*

> *and the registration of voters will be affected as deceased persons must be taken off the voters' roll, which also affects the delimitation of voting districts as well as the arrangements for sick persons that we currently have in place.. ... There will also be an impact on electoral staff especially if we cannot make use of persons who have built up electoral experience. (interview, Hendrickse).*

There is thus a growing awareness that the IEC needs to factor in the various impacts of the epidemic into its strategic planning for how to best fulfil its mandate in future elections (interview, Sampson). What we have not seen yet, however, which is a cause for concern, is that none of this awareness seems to have materialised in terms of strategic planning about how IEC policies, budgets, training and research need to be adjusted. We trust that the awareness expressed by some of the senior staff we talked to in the course of this research will indeed generate a process of reform to further strengthen the IEC's ability to fulfil its mandate despite the problematic consequences of the HIV/AIDS epidemic among the South African electorate.

CONCLUSION

In *Managing HIV/AIDS in the Workplace: A Guide for Government Departments* it is argued that there are four reasons why government departments in particular should respond to the impact of HIV on their work:

- Unless managed HIV and AIDS will make it difficult to achieve the government's transformation goals;
- The Constitution provides that the public service must use resources "efficiently, economically and effectively";
- An integrated HIV/AIDS response will promote confidence in the public service; and
- Responding to HIV/AIDS shows the commitment of the public service to fairness, equity and compassion (Barret Grant, Strode & Smart, 2001).

It is uncontroversial that HIV/AIDS will have an impact on the administration of elections in South Africa. What is more complex is determining the exact nature of this impact and finding ways to mitigate such an impact. Furthermore, unless the IEC itself makes a commitment to address the internal and external impact of HIV/AIDS very little progress will be made. It will be insufficient for the IEC to simply state that it is not stopping people with HIV or AIDS from voting; the bigger question is what is it doing to ensure that such a significant proportion of the population can vote.

The ANC spoke in the same vein about the negative impact on the party of the loss of unique individuals: 'we have lost quite a lot of corporate and intellectual memory of the organisation, of its functioning and policies, to AIDS' (interview, Kariem).

Chapter 6

Impact on Political Parties and Policy Proposals

6.1 Introduction

We have argued above that the election process lies at the core of democracy. It is during this process and on the actual day of elections that the representative nature of the democratic political system is most clearly expressed: politicians ask for the mandate to represent constituencies on the basis of certain policies and the voter decides which candidate or party s/he will entrust with her/his vote after carefully considering the alternatives – at least in theory. In some instances this exchange takes the unusual form of direct one-on-one communication between elites and grassroots.

Arguably the most striking feature of the 2004 election campaign was how President Thabo Mbeki re-connected with ordinary people during his electioneering walkabouts. Had one of those journeys taken him to a township AIDS clinic he most certainly would have been able to skilfully deflect any criticism by pointing to the international praise his government's overall policy programme on HIV and AIDS has received. Had anyone questioned his leadership he would have cited the many thousands of AIDS sufferers who will receive treatment through the government's ambitious roll-out plan. Every question would have had an answer, every demand would have been promised a supply. This is democracy in electioneering mode.

Our point here is not to single out President Mbeki in this regard; no other politician would have acted differently. The imagined encounter at the township AIDS clinic is rather meant to highlight what happened when the issue of HIV/AIDS became an electioneering issue. As such it was simplified and given a party-political "spin" to a degree that voters often were denied a reasonably informed and relevant basis for judging the parties' different proposals on how to address the epidemic. While the issue of HIV/AIDS was by no means special in this regard, few issues needed clear and critical communication more. Having said that, there is little to suggest that a nationwide public debate on HIV/AIDS between contending parties would have altered the election result to a considerable degree – no such public debates, on any issue, were held in the election campaign. Nevertheless it would have gone a long way towards raising people's awareness at a time when their attention was geared towards public political issues. Imagine the effect on public awareness if Mbeki and opposition party leaders Tony Leon, Mangosuthu Buthelezi, Patricia de Lille and Marthinus van Schalkwyk, as well as others in Parliament, had been able to put differences aside and jointly, none before the other, make an appeal for people to avoid infection and not discriminate against those infected – two basic points to which they all ascribe and emphasised in their respective election manifestos. The fact that this did not happen is to a large degree the result of the deep distrust that we found between parties and party leaders on the issue of HIV/AIDS.

Apart from exploring the reasons for and nature of this distrust further, this chapter will analyse some differences in the policy proposals that the parties offered the voters in the 2004 elections and, finally, how the epidemic impacted on the parties' ability to campaign and how the parties, as crucial institutional players in the South African democracy, have prepared internally to meet the challenges that the epidemic presents.

6.2 DEVELOPING POLICIES AND INSTITUTIONS 1992-2004

The reason for the mistrust between the parties on the issue of HIV/AIDS can to a considerable extent be traced back to the various policies and institutional arrangements that have been set in place by the government since 1994, with its many controversial statements of a more rhetorical nature. The brief review that follows here seeks to capture the more critical junctures in this process.[18]

It was noted in chapter two that extraordinary leadership qualities are required from the political establishment to put HIV/AIDS on the political agenda at an early stage in the epidemic, when the disastrous effects of AIDS are not yet noticeable on a larger scale.

This kind of leadership was indeed provided by the ANC and the pre-transition National Party government's Department of Health when they jointly convened a conference on the issue in 1992 that was attended by a large number of actors from the health sector, academic institutions and civil society. The conference was not only about mobilising a political response against HIV/AIDS, but also about establishing a humanitarian and human rights-based approach to those who had been infected, as opposed to the previous largely prejudiced response from the then-National Party government. The conference resulted in the establishment of the National AIDS Committee of South Africa (Nacosa), an umbrella organisation tasked with co-ordinating responses from the state and civil society. However, after publishing an "AIDS Plan" that was well received by stakeholders, the momentum was lost in the political turmoil of the time: "[Whatever] the reason," notes Nattrass, "it is clear that the transitional period of the early 1990s was not a conducive environment for addressing AIDS and contributed to the rapid spread of HIV" (2004:43).

When the ANC-led Government of National Unity (GNU) took office after the 1994 elections, the government adopted the plan that had been formulated by Nacosa as a basis for government policy. The further development and effective implementation of this plan was, however, delayed and made impossible by a number of structural and institutional factors. For instance, a severe shortage of skilled personnel in provincial level government and administration left available funding unused and the positioning of HIV/AIDS policy within the Department of Health effectively narrowed the perception down to the epidemic being a medical problem without further ramifications for society.

Two particularly highly profiled political mistakes added to these problems: the scandal surrounding the musical, *Sarafina II*, and the political support given to Virodene, a product developed by South African researchers that was said to provide the cure against AIDS. While the first scandal revolved both around financial mismanagement and the controversial content of the musical, the second was a case of scientists pulling the wool over politicians' eyes about the nature and effectiveness of a drug they hoped would win themselves international recognition. For the politicians Virodene seemed like a quick-fix solution that would be a panacea against the epidemic. Though different in these regards, both cases represent government efforts to bypass central principles and institutional checks – in the party as well as in the state – that are there to ensure good governance. The government lost credibility in the process, but these scandals also undermined the whole HIV/AIDS sector within civil society, sowing further confusion about the government's commitment to address HIV/AIDS in accordance with policy declarations that would ensure all stakeholders worked together towards a common goal.

Despite these problems, there was as yet no indication that the government's basic understanding of the cause of AIDS departed from that held by mainstream medical research. Calling on South Africans to take personal responsibility to remain uninfected, then-Deputy President Thabo Mbeki said in 1998:

> *For many years, we have allowed the HIV virus [sic] to spread ... [and now] we face the danger that half of our youth will not reach adulthood. Their education will be wasted. The economy will shrink. There will be a large number of sick people whom the healthy will not be able to maintain. Our dreams as a people will be shattered (Cited in Shisana & Zungu-Dirwayi 2003:173).*

This emphasis was at first also expressed by President Mbeki's new cabinet after the 1999 elections, including his Minster of Health, Manto Tshabalala-Msimang. But during the course of 1999, the government incrementally changed its message on the epidemic to the point of appearing to fully embrace the dissident position that HIV does not cause AIDS and, consequently, that ARV treatment is ineffective and harmful. In defending this position President Mbeki addressed a number of international political leaders and organisations in a letter in April 2000:

> *We are now being asked to do precisely the same thing that the racist apartheid tyranny we opposed did, because, it is said, there exists a scientific view that is supported by the majority, against which dissent is prohibited. ... The day may not be far off when we will, once again, see books burnt and their authors immolated by fire by those who believe that they have a duty to conduct a holy crusade against the infidels (Cited in Shisana & Zungu-Dirwayi 2003: 182-3).*

A number of statements to this effect by President Mbeki and Minister Tshabalala-Msimang brought relations between the government and its critics to an all-time low. In direct opposition to the national government the two provincial non-ANC governments, run by the Democratic Alliance in the Western Cape and the Inkatha Freedom Party in KwaZulu-Natal, both announced their intentions to start providing free ARV treatment to pregnant women so as to prevent their children from being infected at birth. These initiatives also had political ramifications within the ANC. Although the ANC as such did not run the Western Cape provincial government at this time, two of the ANC's most senior political figureheads in the province, both with particular responsibilities for developing and implementing ANC health policy, were deeply involved in initiating and running the treatment campaign, for which they received much criticism from some within the leadership of the ANC (interview, Kariem).

There also was much opposition from civil society organisations throughout the country, often spearheaded by the activism of the Treatment Action Campaign (TAC). Launched in 1998 to campaign for free ARV treatment through the public health care system, the TAC laid a charge against the government with the Constitutional Court, arguing that the government failed to live up to its constitutional commitments by not providing treatment. Its greatest victory against the government came when the Court ordered the government to start providing nevirapine to pregnant women to reduce the risk of mother-to-child-transmission at birth. The implementation of this order has been marked by delays and was not fully realised when, in July 2004, the government stated it would no longer recommend Nevirapine as a single therapy medication.

In January 2000 the South African government launched its new institutional initiative to focus and co-ordinate interventions against the epidemic. On the one hand the South African National AIDS Council (Sanac) showed that the government put new emphasis on fighting the epidemic by addressing it as a comprehensive developmental problem beyond the scope of the health ministry and by making the Deputy President its chair. But, on the other hand, it soon became obvious that the council would not become the engine for effective political intervention against the epidemic that had been the intention. Subsequent evaluations of Sanac have found it wanting in the degree to which it was representative, transparent, accountable and efficient (Strode and Barrett Grant, 2004), deficiencies that motivated its reform into a "new" Sanac in early 2004.

The controversies surrounding HIV/AIDS were further compounded in early 2000 with President Mbeki's announcement of the creation of an advisory panel of 33 international AIDS experts, half of whom were so-called dissident researchers, eg researchers who deny that HIV causes AIDS or that HIV even exists. One of the briefs of the panel was to identify – "once and for all" – the scientific evidence of the cause of AIDS. However, the work of the panel was fraught with tension and distrust between mainstream and dissident researchers, with the former arguing that this evidence was already at hand, a claim that was not accepted by the latter group (Schoofs, 2000). The work of the panel, as it was constituted originally, came to an end in April 2001 with the presentation of a report that contained two separate and contradictory lists of recommendations, one from each group of researchers. In responding to the report Health Minister Tshabalala-Msimang said that the government's approach would remain "rooted in the premise that HIV causes AIDS" (cited in Van der Vliet, 2004: 62). To the government's critics the panel had been a waste of time and resources that had sowed immense confusion among people and had thus undermined much of the HIV/AIDS awareness that had been generated by grassroots activists and NGOs for a number of years.

However, parallel to approaching the dissident position in many of its statements and being told by the Constitutional Court how to prioritise its resources in combating the epidemic, the government had been working on developing a comprehensive overall policy framework since July 1999. The policy document, *HIV/AIDS & STD: Strategic Plan for South Africa 2000-2005*, was launched in early 2000 and soon received much praise by many world leaders for being one of the best in the developing world. Not only did it elevate the fight against HIV/AIDS institutionally in government and state structures through Sanac, but it also sought to include civil society in a partnership to pool resources in the fight against HIV/AIDS. All was well on the level of policy formulation. However, the implementation of the policy would soon be found wanting, partly because of the problems with Sanac that were noted above and partly because of a lack of human resources and skills in the public health care system, as well as more institutional and structural resources. While this no doubt is true, the relevant point here is that the government, despite having placed its overall policy within the paradigm of mainstream research, continually undermined its own statements by communicating – intentionally or not – perceptions and convictions that undermined the very foundations of its elaborate policy intentions (Van der Vliet, 2004).

The government's most recent major policy announcement was made in November 2003 when it declared that it would launch a large-scale roll-out of free ARV treatment through the public health care system. This was a change in policy since the government previously had declared that such an ambitious programme would be too expensive or impossible for reasons such as a lack of capacity. The government explained its shift in policy by a sharp drop in the price of medication and a phasing-in approach to the treatment where capacity exists. The first deadline that the government set for itself was to deliver treatment to 53 000 people by March 2004. The announcement was met with much jubilation from the government's critics but, as with previous ambitious policies, this has been marked by delays and deadlines have been pushed into the future. At the deadline for this report up to 11 200 South Africans were receiving medication through the programme (Business Day 28 October 2004). We shall see below how these delays and the way that the treatment programme was announced have fuelled distrust of the government's intentions from some of its parliamentary critics.

6.3 POLITICAL PARTIES ON HIV/AIDS AND ELECTIONS

Given the magnitude of the epidemic and the fact that it has a potential to reach into virtually all spheres of private and public life and given that so far the political response has been ambiguous to say the least, it would not have been surprising if one of the political parties contesting the election had, perhaps, been the Positive Party. As a "single-issue" party propagating AIDS awareness, prevention and treatment it would not really have contested elections with an ambition to win control of government. Its mandate from the voters would rather have been to ensure that the epidemic is never sidelined in the legislative work of Parliament. Our point here is just to highlight the fact that despite the relatively low threshold for launching a party – in essence R500, 50 signatures and a logo – this obviously was not considered a viable and effective strategy by AIDS activists in the run-up to the 2004 elections. There would, no doubt, have been many obstacles to such a party actually winning seats in Parliament, but, arguably, it would by no means have been impossible to win the necessary roughly 30 000 seats needed to guarantee AIDS activism a parliamentary platform.

This is not to suggest that such a strategy would not be problematic for various reasons, only to highlight that it has been a possible route that has not (yet?) been chosen.

As we now shall explore how the epidemic has affected the political parties in the 2004 elections campaign we will organise our discussion under four headings that capture different aspects of this possible effect. The electioneering material was gathered from all the parties that had representation in the National Assembly prior to the 2004 elections. This was followed up with interviews with representatives of the biggest parties – the African National Congress (ANC), the Democratic Alliance (DA) and the Inkatha Freedom Party (IFP) – and the smaller parties that had given the issue of HIV/AIDS particular emphasis in their campaign and manifestoes – the Independent Democrats (ID), the New National Party (NNP) and the African Christian Democratic Party (ACDP).

6.3.1 INTEGRITY OF THE ELECTION

We saw in the chapter on governance that scholars hypothesise that the integrity and legitimacy of elections might be undermined if the epidemic reduces the capacity of the electoral commission and the accuracy of the voters' roll. This fear, however, was in general not reflected by the representatives of the political parties. The argument that the epidemic impacted on the election outcome could have been made more convincingly, argued the NNP's Kobus Gous, if the election had been a "close race", but with the dominance of the ANC this effect was negligible. Other representatives agreed and one added that it was likely to become a much greater problem in running the next general election in

2009. In general all but one representative assumed that the IEC had been able to mobilise all the necessary staff and that the voters' roll was as accurate as it possibly could be. It seemed that the scenario of the epidemic affecting the capacity of the IEC, thus possibly undermining the legitimacy of the electoral process, has not really been considered by the different parties.

The one exception to this which expressed trust and confidence in the IEC was the IFP, which at one stage threatened to lodge a formal complaint against the ANC, but for reasons unrelated to the theme of this report.

The IFP's Rabinowitz was however also critical of the IEC for failing to ensure that a sufficient number of fully equipped and staffed voting stations had been in place to guarantee people the chance to vote in more distant rural areas. This was coupled with the party noting that the "special vote" was not made use of effectively at all in KwaZulu-Natal (interview, Rabinowitz). This specific criticism of the weak realisation of the "special vote" was not solely expressed by the IFP. The ANC's Saadiq Kariem also spoke of the many hospitalised voters who had never been informed properly about the special vote: "It did not work well in hospitals. It could have been much better," (interview, Kariem). The special vote, argued Kariem, is exactly the kind of institutional arrangement that is necessary to protect the right to vote of those who are ill, be it from AIDS or not, but many more resources and effort are need to actually realise this commitment.

6.3.2 PARTY CAPACITY TO CAMPAIGN

Political parties rely heavily on their many supporters at the time of elections. The level of mass support for a party does not matter in the least if it does not transfer into active casting of votes for the party on the day of elections (voter participation will be explored further in chapter seven). But the other instance when a strong and well-mobilised support base is necessary is during the election campaign. A party that has had its capacity to launch and sustain an effective election campaign undermined for some reason will suffer for it at the polls. Since this ability to a large extent hinges on the strong and active mobilisation of party cadres, including those in the many local branches far from the national scene, their reduced capacity to work in the campaign as a direct or indirect consequence of AIDS will aggregate into a weaker campaign overall.

The IFP spoke of an increased need to replace party cadres due to AIDS-related illnesses or death. While this caused some strain on party structures and on its ability to campaign, the regular processes for such replacements were still functioning on the whole. The party did not experience any "gaps" in its organisational structures for this reason, but the loss of seniority and experience nevertheless reduced the party's capacity somewhat (interview, Rabinowitz).

The ANC spoke in the same vein about the negative impact on the party of the loss of unique individuals: "We have lost quite a lot of corporate and intellectual memory of the organisation, of its functioning and policies, to AIDS" (interview, Kariem). A more indirect effect of AIDS on party capacity in the campaign was reported by the ACDP. As a party explicitly based on Christian principles the ACDP has many pastors in leadership positions throughout its national and provincial structures. These senior party representatives were unable to participate in many regular Saturday election rallies as they were called on to officiate over an unprecedented number of funerals in their respective congregations (interview, Dudley).

This effect on party capacity will of course be reduced with the availability of ARV treatment. While all parties have comprehensive medical schemes for their leaders and representatives at national and provincial levels that provide full access to ARV medication, the same cannot be said for all local level representatives and party workers more generally. For the ANC, however, this had not merely been an issue of internal capacity. Saadiq Kariem elaborated on the policy implications of the fact that "quite a number of parliamentarians are [HIV] positive and are on treatment", as well as that all the medical schemes that the ANC offers its employees provide full coverage ARV treatment:

> *I think that's also why so many of the grassroots, the ordinary membership, felt so strongly about antiretrovirals because if treatment was good for some in the organisation, obviously that same policy has to be good for everybody else. That is why there was so much anger at the dithering of everybody on the policy issue (interview, Kariem).*

While no party reported a major impact of the epidemic on its capacity to campaign effectively, it seems clear that such effects are beginning to be felt by some. How strong this negative impact on a party is will depend largely on the extent of its support in the population, as well as on whether its main constituency overlaps with the groups in the population that are particularly affected by the epidemic. The effect in this regard is of course not predetermined but can be reduced at least to some extent by what practices the party has institutionalised in response to the epidemic. The responses reviewed in the section below, however, leave much to be desired on that score.

6.3.3 PARTY PRACTICE

According to one train of thought, democracy is and should be an institutionalised competition between elites for power on the basis of their support among the electorate. In this elitist interpretation of democracy political parties are mainly campaign vehicles with the sole purpose of maximising the vote and propelling elites into office. Since parties have no more general value they need not ascribe to any particular principles of good governance as long as they produce the intended result; parties need not be democratic in themselves. A close approximation of this general description is the Democratic and Republican parties in the United States. A more community-oriented political party culture has its origins in Western Europe. In this tradition political parties are very much part of the web of more or less political associations that continually inform, shape and help formulate people's social and political priorities, identities and interactions. The close ties between Social Democratic parties and trade unions, and between Christian Democratic parties and religious congregations, are perhaps the clearest examples of how such parties are woven into the social fabric of communities. According to this interpretation, political parties should be "schools of democracy" with internal structures, practices and values that mirror those it would like to see in the whole of society.

These opposing political party traditions have different implications when, as in South Africa, much of the social and political discourse is dominated by the HIV/AIDS epidemic. In the elitist interpretation there is no need for a political party to internalise the implications of the epidemic into its party structures and culture. If a party official or volunteer is affected by the epidemic they would be expected to seek redress outside party structures – the way that the party deals with the epidemic has no bearing on its proposed HIV/AIDS policy if elected into government. However, as a "school of democracy", a political party would be expected to reflect the caring community that it – presumably – wishes to create for the whole of society as a means to combat the epidemic. As such the party would provide or facilitate access to counselling and treatment and its leaders would seek actively to break down stigma through various public initiatives that challenge the prejudices connected with the epidemic.

On the whole the credibility of the party's promised HIV/AIDS policies for the nation would be undermined if the party did not have a track record of living by those policies on a small scale within its own "party-community".

While it would take comprehensive research to authoritatively apply this general outline of party political cultures to South Africa, our understanding of the political parties in South Africa is that they all, more or less, are or seek to become an integral part of community life in South Africa. None is explicitly elitist and some have a very ambitious vision of permeating civil society, an ambition that might be problematic in itself. The only more general normative point we will make is that to the extent we are right in saying all parties to some degree lean towards being community oriented, they should be criticised if this ambition is not reflected in how they internally approach and deal with the implications of the epidemic. Our normative argument is that a party that seeks to be a "school of democracy" in the sense we discuss here needs to implement democratic governance on HIV/AIDS within its own structures to be a fully credible political force for a progressive and comprehensive political response to the epidemic.

The responses we got from the parties to our questions on party practice generate the general picture that they all fall short on this score. No party has institutionalised a response in the sense that the party has identified a process whereby a member can seek support and assistance on learning they are HIV positive. The representatives of the ACDP, ANC, ID and IFP all told of one or more instances when a party colleague had experienced an HIV-related crisis – either learning they were HIV positive or falling ill from an AIDS-related illness – and they all claimed that the party or individual party colleagues did provide some support. But on probing this with the representatives it became clear that this support had been given on an ad hoc basis and that the nature of the support to some extent depended on the seniority and/or well-connectedness of the party colleague. That is to say that the support that was provided was not based on a policy and an institutionalised process; neither was it conceived of as a right to which the party had identified a reciprocal commitment.

Although the representatives we spoke to were all the spokespersons on HIV/AIDS for their respective parties, none had been identified by his/her party as the person that party members should turn to with personal concerns relating to the epidemic; no party had identified such a person at all.

Also the question of how the party leadership reflected the issue within the party left much to be desired, albeit that the responses were more diversified in this regard. With the sole exception of the leadership of the ID, no party leadership had spearheaded a campaign for members to take an HIV test by publicly taking one themselves. Cheryllyn Dudley (ACDP) had done a test in the morning of our interview and spoke of how doing so had opened her eyes to the stigma that is attached to the test itself. She, as well as the DA's Mike Waters, said they naturally included their various personal experiences and reflections upon taking the test in their respective campaign speeches, thus personalising the issue with the intention of breaking down prejudiced perceptions of the test. The NNP's Kobus Gous said he too would do the same when he was convinced it served an actual purpose and was not only a form of political rhetoric. Saadiq Kariem of the ANC elaborated on the fact that the positions held by party leadership about taking the test and the epidemic more generally did not accurately represent the party:

> *I get approached regularly by ordinary party members and some Parliament members who are HIV positive and need treatment or some form of advice. I think there is a lot more acceptance among rank and file, and there is a lot more awareness and openness. It is unfortunate that some of the leaders have come out so strongly publicly by saying that they are not aware of people with HIV/AIDS. But among the rank and file there is a lot more acceptance. The perception that the public get by statements that the leadership make are actually different from what is happening among rank and file membership (interview, Kariem).*

It is not our intention here to pass moral judgement in any way on any individual, be it a political leader or not, for what s/he decides in terms of publicly announcing an HIV test. There are, naturally, immensely personal considerations that have to be respected. Our comment though is that the epidemic places new demands of a more personal nature on a person who wants to be a constructive role-model in the fight against the epidemic by her/his own actions – political leadership in the context of the epidemic is as difficult as that!

The resignation from government of the leader of the IFP, Mangosuthu Buthelezi, after the election in April 2004 seems to have enabled him to be more outspoken and critical on the issue of HIV/AIDS. While he has tried to raise awareness about the epidemic in his KwaZulu-Natal constituency for a number of years (interview, Rabinowitz), the decision to speak critically on the national scene was triggered by the tragic loss of two of his children to AIDS-related illnesses shortly after the April elections. Just the mere public recognition by Buthelezi of the true cause of death of his children was important as it was, to our knowledge, the first time a South African politician of that stature personalised the effects of the epidemic so dramatically.

Although presumably the most painful, these deaths in his family were not the first time Dr Buthelezi came into direct contact with AIDS. In a thinly veiled criticism of President Mbeki's statement that he knows of no one who has died from AIDS, the IFP's Ruth Rabinowitz said: "Buthelezi knows many HIV-positive people and many who have died from AIDS" (interview, Rabinowitz). On a superficial level it might seem paradoxical that the political leader who has been the strongest proponent of merging the conservative Zulu ethnic culture and its institutions with the new democratic South Africa should be the leader who identifies himself most personally with an issue as controversial as the epidemic. Indeed, as we review the discussions in our focus group interviews in chapter ten, we shall see, in stark colours, how problematic that cultural paradigm is for people who are directly affected by or infected with the epidemic. But if one goes beyond the apparent contradictions, argued Rabinowitz, the dual leadership mandate held by Buthelezi – as the leader of a "modern" political party and as a traditional leader of Zulu loyalists – places a special responsibility on him to address the hardships of his community in a personal capacity. Although very important and impressive, Buthelezi's leadership profile on HIV/AIDS does not seem to have become institutionalised in his party; the IFP's record matches the other parties in this regard.

In mid-October 2004 the DA adopted a proposal by its new spokesperson on health, MP Ryan Coetzee, which has the potential to address the shortcomings we noted in the DA's internal response to the epidemic. Under the heading, Leading by example – a DA HIV/AIDS campaign, the policy sets out what "strong leadership" should mean for the DA in the context of the epidemic. The proposal means, in essence, that every DA representative must show stronger leadership by leading by example in terms of talking openly about the epidemic but also preferably by publicly getting tested for HIV. About a month later, on 12 November 2004, the media reported how most of the DA's national leadership took public HIV tests as part of the party's HIV/AIDS awareness campaign.

It is the ID, which stands out as the party that has done the most work on how to build a party, that in itself – in its structures, policies and internal party culture – seeks to address the epidemic in various ways. In one sense this is very impressive, but it would be hard to imagine starting a new party with a progressive agenda in present-day South Africa that did not set its focus on the epidemic. Unlike other parliamentary parties the ID did not have to incrementally adjust its policies to try to bring its established constituency along on an ever-stronger response to a worsening epidemic. Unlike other parties for which the resulting policies are more or less sustainable compromises between competing moral and human right-based paradigms, as well as between contending representatives for alternative budget posts, the ID could formulate its policies and decide on strategies with a relatively clean slate. This is not to suggest that members and leaders of the ID have not debated and at times differed on policies and strategies (interview, Greyling), but that this has been less of a concern than for other parties.

Until the November 2004 initiative from the DA it was, to the best of our knowledge, the leader of the ID, Patricia de Lille, who was the only party leader to have publicly announced taking an HIV test. Her example was subsequently followed by the ID's nine provincial leaders. In another equally important policy, the party has decided to nominate at least one openly HIV-positive member for a parliamentary seat. Well aware of the risks of that person becoming merely a "token" for the issue, Greyling spoke about the need for that person to be a strong member of the party with all the right qualifications for taking a parliamentary seat, over and above being able to speak on the issue of HIV/AIDS with an immediate personal experience of the epidemic.

At the time seats won in the 2004 elections were distributed to members on the party list there was indeed a candidate with those qualifications. However, after a process of consultation, the member and the party finally agreed to go along with her doctor's advice that she should not take up the seat due to the high work load and stress of the job (interview, Greyling).

In its different initiatives to provide leadership and representation in addressing the epidemic the ID has pushed the boundaries of what it is possible to accomplish in the parliamentary arena. In part because of these initiatives, argued Greyling, members speak openly and without fear of stigma within the party about how the epidemic is impacting on their lives; but the party has nevertheless not institutionalised a channel of support where privacy is ensured in case this was preferred by a party member. Personal details aside, the lessons learned by the ID's effort to nominate a party candidate to a parliamentary seat arguably suggests a point of general relevance. As is the case in the discourse on the merits and problems of affirmative action more broadly, it is important that a person who gets nominated to a parliamentary seat at least in part because she is HIV positive gets the necessary backup, both from the party, but also from Parliament itself. It is important to remember that such an MP would not be the only HIV-positive MP in Parliament. But while other infected MPs can hide their potential problems in fulfilling all aspects of the workload behind various explanations, any such deficiency with the MP who is openly positive is likely to be reduced to his/her HIV status, whether this is true or not. For it to become a viable option for any one individual to function effectively as an MP, despite being openly HIV positive it is imperative that Parliament recognises HIV infection as a disability that allows the MP whatever s/he needs to enable her/him to function through the various stages of her/his disease. In his brief response to our inquiry about what support parliament provides in this regard, the then-Secretary of Parliament, S Mfenyana, responded that Parliament does not have any knowledge of the HIV status of MPs. If an MP decides to disclose his/her HIV-positive status, parliament would provide professional counselling and advice on medical matters.

As Parliament does not provide MPs with a medical aid scheme of its own, MPs are required to choose a scheme that best suits their needs. Mfenyana continues:

> *Parliament's Human Resources section is currently drafting a policy on HIV and AIDS in the workplace. The policy will address issues of labour*

> *relations and conditions of service with regard to employees affected by HIV and AIDS, infected with HIV and/or suffering from AIDS-related diseases (letter dated 1 April 2004).*

Our interpretation of the information provided by Mfenyana is that Parliament is busy addressing the implications of the epidemic for its employed staff, which of course is a very important step in the right direction, but there is nothing to suggest that Parliament is considering what institutional and other arrangements might be necessary to enable HIV-positive MPs to work effectively in the political legislature after publicly announcing their HIV status.

6.3.4 POLICY PROPOSALS

Much pre-election news commentary on the various parties' policy proposals in the election campaign noted their many similarities on most issues and on HIV/AIDS in particular. This is correct in that all parties suggested a combination of political interventions to prevent further infections, treat those who are suffering from AIDS and ensure that they are not discriminated against, and to care for those affected by the epidemic, especially the orphans. While a careful perusal of the documents will indicate that the parties balance the different interventions somewhat differently in their overall response, there are a few stark differences in what the parties offered the voters. The political representatives concur with this observation. "The difficulty I had in pre-election debates where I was pitted against a DA person," says the ANC's Saadiq Kariem, "was that we were saying the same things" (interview, Kariem). The NNP's Kobus Gous agreed: "Parties are in agreement on 95% on what should be the political response to the epidemic, so it should disappear as a political issue. It should – but it will not" (interview, Gous).

One of the reasons why it will not disappear is that it matters to people, which is why political parties would focus their campaigning on the remaining 5% of policy differences to see if this could win them additional votes. Another reason why HIV/AIDS will not disappear as a political issue is that, despite the many similarities on a policy level, there are wide differences on a level of principle. It is, arguably, only by analysing this level of the politics of HIV/AIDS in South Africa that we can begin to understand why it generates such intense "political heat". Our discussion is based on the main election manifestos and any other material generated by the parties for the explicit purpose of informing the public about their respective policies on dealing with HIV/AIDS as part of the election campaign, as well as on our interviews with party representatives.[19]

Our suggestion here is to analyse the various parties' policy positions on HIV/AIDS along two dimensions on the level of principle: the first is whether the political response should be based within a human rights approach, and the second is whether the political response should be directed at the infected individual or the affected community. The four different possible policy options that this analytical scheme generates are presented in table 24 together with our interpretation of how the different parties should be placed along the two dimensions.

Table 24. Two dimensions to HIV/AIDS policy

		Human rights approach	
		yes	no
Focus of policy	individual	ANC, DA, ID	NNP
	community	IFP	ACDP

Any analytical effort such as this naturally represents a simplification of complexities and insensitivity to nuances, but this is not a problem as long as it helps us to clarify correctly some more fundamental aspects of reality that the many details otherwise blind us to. Our discussion in this section will seek to motivate our positioning of the different parties in relation to the two principles.

To take a human rights approach to HIV/AIDS is to argue that the political intervention against the epidemic should be based on a commitment to respect and realise a set of human rights even if this runs counter to public sentiment or political expediency (Heywood, 2000). Advocates of this approach might argue the relevance of different sets of human rights, either those defined by the 1948 United Nations Charter of Fundamental Human Rights or any more recent national equivalent. The South African Constitution provides unusually strong assistance for this argument; not only is it exceptionally liberal in awarding a wide set of human rights, but it also makes socioeconomic rights legally binding on the state, albeit under certain conditions. The ANC, DA, IFP and ID are clear in their commitments towards these rights. There is a nuance in the IFP's policies, however, than motivates it being identified as focusing its policies on the community and not the individual. The human rights approach in dealing with the epidemic must shift, argued the IFP's Ruth Rabinowitz, from focusing on the individual's right to privacy and integrity to his/her right to non-discrimination from the community. The policy is thus community centred in that it will seek to create caring communities in which individuals who are known to be HIV positive are taken care of and respected nevertheless.

It is the ACDP that most strongly objects to the human rights approach. In arguing for a political intervention that is based on the ACDP's formulation of Christian values, Cheryllyn Dudley criticised the ANC for treating HIV/AIDS:

> *...purely as a human rights issue and not as a contagious disease. Our understanding is that if it is going to be contained and dealt with it is going to have to be treated as a contagious disease. We can't just wish it away. With the best will in the world, lighting candles and wearing ribbons until we are blue in the face will just not do it (interview, Dudley).*

From this understanding flows the ACDP's proposal to make HIV testing compulsory and HIV infection notifiable. On balance, the human rights of the individual must not be allowed to obstruct effective political interventions to combat the epidemic.

The NNP's Kobus Gous agrees that the human rights approach is problematic:

> *By emphasising the HR approach to the epidemic we have emphasised the stigma that we inherited from Western Europe and the US where it was*

> *primarily a homosexual disease. In Africa where the epidemic is not linked to homosexuality we are perpetuating this "homosexual agenda" by elevating the disease as a human rights issue. Whereas if you treat it as simply another disease the stigma would have disappeared by now, as it did in relation to TB and other diseases. We are actually perpetuating the stigma by emphasising the HR aspects of the epidemic. Such rights are guaranteed anyway on an individual basis, so why make such an issue out of it (interview, Gous).*

While it differs from the ACDP stand, this position does not lead the NNP to argue for making HIV or AIDS notifiable, albeit for pragmatic and not principled reasons, since the NNP argues such measures would be ineffective and counterproductive (interview, Gous). In our understanding the ACDP and the NNP also differ on their more fundamental reason for challenging the human rights agenda. Whereas the NNP argues pragmatically that it "perpetuates the stigma," the ACDP's objection is based on the party's moral convictions. Its election manifesto makes it clear that inappropriately explicit sex education for children coupled with the availability of contraceptives represent "moral degeneration" in South Africa. This moral degeneration also has had a direct impact on the epidemic. The party programme argues that "the unprecedented moral degeneration in the country over the past ten years of democracy has resulted in dysfunctional families, widespread crime and corruption and the spread of the HIV/Aids pandemic" (ACDP 2004). The proposed link between homosexuality and the human rights approach was elaborated on by Dudley in criticising the DA's policies for being even more problematic in terms of their human rights approach:

> *They [the DA] are "big talk" now about various issues, but when it comes down to it, nothing will get done because of their "super-liberal" policies. ... For a long time we have realised that the DA are strongly motivated in terms of the gay agenda (interview, Dudley).*

The ACDP's policy can be summarised as arguing that to effectively combat the epidemic, political intervention is needed that infringes on the individual's right to privacy and integrity, and his/her right to sexual preference, for the sake of the (as yet uninfected) community. The fundamental reason for this, however, is not the rights of the individual members of the community to remain uninfected, but the reinvigoration that such policies would represent of the ACDP's formulation of Christian morals.

Our brief analysis in this section has emphasised two differences on a level of principles that we could identify after reading election material and interviewing party representatives. The result contradicts the perception that the parties, by and large, offer the same policy proposals and that differences can be found only in the details and not in kind. On the contrary, we found the human rights dimension to be a particularly clear dividing line between some of the parties. However, as our analysis of the campaign strategies will show in the next section, parties that embraced the same combination of principles still had many grounds for disagreement and mistrust.

6.3.5 HIV/AIDS AS A CAMPAIGN ISSUE IN 2004

Our questions to the party representatives about how the HIV/AIDS issue had been used in the election campaign generated some strong views that at time boarded on frustration and anger; a testimony to the emotions and fundamental values into which the issue taps. Before we report these comments, however, it is important to note that whether or not the issue of HIV/AIDS should feature at all as an electioneering issue is far from obvious. Where this is the case, particularly in the context of a developing country in the grip of the epidemic, the democratic system becomes vulnerable to the populism of political entrepreneurs who promise quick and simple solutions to complex problems. The alternative would be to form a "policy accord" between all of the largest parties contesting the elections; Botswana and Tanzania are good examples in this regard where the parliamentary parties have institutionalised a common response to the epidemic.[20] Such a strategy would reduce the risk of populism taking hold and thus ensure some stability and long-term vision on the agreed-upon political intervention against the epidemic. All party representatives argued that they ideally would have preferred not to campaign on the HIV/AIDS issue, but that they wished instead that all parties had agreed to a comprehensive policy accord that was certain to be effective against the epidemic. This had happened a number of years ago. However, such an agreement would be sound and constructive only if the policy that the parties agreed upon was strong with a realistic chance to tackle the epidemic – something that cannot be assumed. Dudley of the ACDP elaborated on the importance of politicising the issue in the election campaign:

> *The government's U-turn would not have happened without pressure from opposition parties, but civil society lobby groups such as the TAC as well as the court cases must also get credit; all of this has been continuing for some time. However, nothing will work like the election time. It would therefore have been cruel and wicked for us to have negotiated to keep it off the election agenda, leaving people behind, instead of pressuring government to do the right thing (interview, Dudley).*

This point is potentially critically important more generally for the legitimacy of the democratic system as such since, by removing the issue from the election campaign, the parties would have made it much more difficult for the voters to hold the parties accountable for poorly devised or ineffectively implemented policy interventions.

Given that HIV/AIDS was an electioneering issue, what strategic role did it play in the campaign? It is easy to imagine that if the ANC had not changed its policy in November 2003 to launch a treatment roll-out, the party would have been very vulnerable to critique on this point in the campaign (Willan, 2004). To the opposition parties we talked to there was no doubt at all that the change in policy, and the timing of that change, can be explained by the success of ANC election strategists in convincing the party leadership that this would be necessary to stop a haemorrhaging of party support at the polls. The argument was made most strongly by Dudley:

I think in this last year they have realised the seriously negative impact that their behaviour has had and so the roll-out has been held back purposely to be a gift from "ANC-God" at this hour, and because it is such a life and death thing that is so close to people's hearts I really think that they may well have succeeded with that strategy It is sad (interview, Dudley).

Mike Waters of the DA agreed that the issue was no longer as clear cut as before November 2003, but argued that, since announcing the turnaround, the ANC had made many statements that placed doubts in peoples' minds about its commitment to the programme:

The first promise was that at end of March, 53 000 would be on ARV treatment. They announced in Parliament yesterday [25 February] that this is not going to happen, and they were not prepared to give a date for when it is going to happen. Now, if they are prepared to break their first promise on the eve of a general election, I shudder to think what they are going to do after the election, because they have got nothing to loose after that (interview, Waters).

The opposition strategy was therefore to question the ANC's and especially the minister of health's (and thereby implicitly the president's) commitment to the roll-out.

The ANC's Kariem agreed that HIV/AIDS was problematic for the ANC in the election. It was an issue where the opposition could score points: "if anything the epidemic enhanced their ability to campaign because it was our Achilles heel ... our soft spot" (interview, Kariem). This had become even clearer to the party leadership after a survey among ANC members was conducted in early 2003 in which the ANC's policy on treatment was challenged.[21] He strongly opposed the interpretation, however, that the policy U-turn in November was based on anything less than a full commitment from the ANC or that it had been timed strategically for maximum effect in the election campaign. While the ANC's internal policy survey would have provided important information that would have been useful for strategic purposes, he argued that:

the policy U-turn, if you want to call it that, was more a result of sustained internal pressure over a long time. If the survey hadn't happened [the ANC] would still have gone down the same route. If anything the survey would have added support to what we had been saying for the last four years. It's been a long battle. (interview, Kariem)

The "we" in the quote above refers to those members of the ANC National Health Committee who since 1999 have been advising the ANC political leadership to strengthen and mainstream its approach to the epidemic. "The policy change in November 2003 on ARVs", continued Kariem, "came about as a result of sustained pressure from 1999 to change the mindset, which took several years to get to the point where politically we can now say that we have turned the corner". Kariem's insider analysis is of course immensely helpful for understanding recent developments and shifts in ANC policy on this issue as he offers a glimpse of the political dynamics that are internal to the ANC, a dynamic that comments by opposition representatives do not factor into the analysis at all. It remains to be seen, however, if Kariem is right in saying that the government has "turned the corner" in its policy. Although Kariem's analysis suggests a more complex process of policy-making and multi-dimensional reasons for policy change than those offered by the others we talked to, his comment shares the basic logic with those of the government's critics that it took "sustained pressure" to change the minds of the ANC's top political leadership on the HIV/AIDS issue, it was not an initiative from the top.

CONCLUSION

Our analysis of the way in which the HIV/AIDS epidemic has impacted on the parliamentary parties in South Africa has presented a basic normative position that, to some degree, applies to all parties: they need to lead by example within their own party-community if they want to ensure democratic governance on HIV/AIDS for the whole country. Most parties fell far short of what can be expected in this regard, but there are exceptions. The ID has provided such leadership already and the DA is planning to do the same. While these steps are important within the parties to show the required leadership, there appears to be much more fundamental fault lines of distrust between the parties that for the foreseeable future will make any attempts to unify the parliamentary parties in the fight against the epidemic impossible. While this is the case it would seem futile to even imagine an all-party policy accord on HIV/AIDS for South Africa. Competitive democratic elections, and not cooperation, will provide the incentives for improving the political response to the epidemic.

Part 3

Exploring the Impact on Voter Participation

Those who provide home-based care are somewhat more likely to be members of local development organisations and a great deal more likely to attend community meetings. On the other hand they are somewhat less likely to discuss politics with friends.

Chapter 7

Political Opinion and Participation in the Context of the Epidemic

In Part 2 of the report we discussed the institutional responses that have been set up by the state and/or political parties to meet the challenges posed by the epidemic. In the next four chapters we shall shift our focus to look at the South African electorate. In this chapter we will make use of the Afrobarometer surveys of South Africans' political opinions and degree of political activism. As one in a network of such continental opinion "barometers," the Afrobarometer provides not only information about South Africa, but allows for comparison with countries in sub-Saharan Africa and beyond. The survey data enables us to investigate how people prioritise issues relating to the epidemic and to explore what factors explain why some feel it is more important than others. We also will explore how the epidemic impacts on people's ability to participate in political activities in civil society.

7.1 POLITICAL OPINION ON HIV/AIDS

The first round of the Afrobarometer survey was conducted in nine countries in southern Africa during the course of 1999 and 2000 and the survey contained a few questions that explored people's opinions and experiences in relation to the HIV/AIDS epidemic. In their analysis of this data Alan Whiteside et al report that the attitudinal data from the survey corroborate the epidemiological data; both sources of information indicate that many people in South and southern Africa are very ill and are dying in increasing numbers.

However, a surprising pattern emerges when they probe how people's political priorities relate to the epidemic:

> *[Even] where HIV/AIDS has reached severe levels and people are dying in large and rising numbers, and even where people recognize those deaths as the result of HIV infection, very few of them place HIV/AIDS high on the agenda for government intervention. Rather, the epidemic is superseded in most countries by demands for government action to create jobs, expand the economy, and improve crime and security, or is masked by demands for overall improvements in health-related services (Whiteside et al, 2002:26).*

The authors conclude that this might indeed be a rational response since most people in the region have to endure and try to survive the daily threats to their health caused by poverty, many of which are more direct and visible than HIV infection or even illness and death from AIDS.

A second round of the Afrobarometer survey was conducted in 15 countries in the sub-continent during 2002 and 2003. While the results from this second survey still need to be analysed in further depth, initial analyses indicate a number of potentially important changes. Table 25 shows the percentages of people who thought AIDS was the most important problem facing their government, who thought the government should prioritise the fight against the epidemic, even at the expense of other development-related issues such as education, and who had experienced personal loss in terms of having had a close friend or family member die from an AIDS-related disease.

Table 25. Opinions and experience of the epidemic in sub-Saharan Africa

	AIDS most important problem [A]		Prioritise AIDS [B]	Personal loss from AIDS [C]		Adult HIV prevalence[D]
	2002-2003	1999-2000	2002-2003	2002-2003	1999-2000	End of 2003
Botswana	30	24	47	36	32	37.3
Cabo Verde	2	-	53	12	-	-
Ghana	3	-	35	19	-	3.1
Kenya	10	-	36	66	-	6.7
Lesotho	5	0.5	57	18	11	28.9
Malawi	3	2	47	57	65	14.2
Mali	1	0	46	17	12	1.9
Mozambique	16	-	53	27	-	12.2
Namibia	28	14	35	71	40	21.3
Nigeria	4	-	44	11	-	5.4
Senegal	1	-	44	14	-	0.8
South Africa	26	13	40	18	16	21.5
Tanzania	14	0.5	47	61	60	8.8
Uganda	7	0.5	52	85	-	4.1
Zambia	3	0	33	74	65	16.5

A) Percentage of people who regard AIDS to be the most serious problem facing their country. B) Percentage of people who think the government should spend more resources on AIDS even at the expense of other development issues. C) Percentage of people who have lost one or more friend or relative to AIDS.
Source: A-C) Mattes 2004. D) UNAIDS 2004.

We can see that, with a few exceptions, the epidemic is experienced as a problem by larger sections of the populations than only two or three years earlier. In some instances the increase in public awareness is considerable: twice as many South Africans and Namibians consider it to be the most important problem and the people who have experienced (or admit to having experienced) a personal loss to AIDS rose by up to 70%. The anomaly is the indication that fewer Malawians have experienced personal loss, but otherwise there is an increase across the board (most of which is well over the margin of error of about +/- 2 percentages) suggesting that the epidemic is experienced as an increasingly problematic political and social problem. However, beyond reporting these percentages, there are few consistent patterns between these and other more political variables. In other words, as far as the data have been analysed to this point there is no basis for arguing that the epidemic is shaping political opinion and behaviour in a consistent fashion across the southern African countries.

7.1.1 EXPLAINING POLITICAL OPINION ON THE EPIDEMIC

How people respond to the two explicitly political questions relating to the epidemic that we discussed above – what the person thought of the government's performance on the issue of HIV/AIDS and whether the person would like the government to prioritise spending resources on fighting HIV/AIDS even if this implies less money for education and other development oriented political goals – can potentially have many different explanations that are in themselves more or less linked to the epidemic. The only probable explanation that we found, however, was whether people had had the difficult experience of losing a family member or a close friend to the epidemic, an experience that had a stronger correlation to the second question than to the first question (Pearson's r = .195 at .01 level of significance). When the information was broken down according to race groups, gender and urban or rural setting, some correlations were even stronger.[22] However, to assess the strength of these correlations even further we tested to see if they would remain as strong and significant even after controlling for a person's level of education and household income. This means that we checked that the statistical pattern we observed was not in fact caused by either levels of education or income. The experience of personal loss proved to be a relatively good predictor of a person's opinion on the question, even when the two alternative explanations were taken into account.[23] These results should not really come as a surprise as one can easily imagine the rationale behind a person wanting the government to prioritise AIDS after having been effected in such a direct and tragic way.

We would, however, be mistaken to assume that this prioritisation by people who have suffered personal loss led them to be more critical of the government. When the same statistical analyses were made on the hypothesis that personal loss explains a person's opinion on whether the government has performed well in dealing with the epidemic, the statistical correlations were weaker and less significant across the board. This result seems to indicate that people's frustration with government priorities does not necessarily transform into an outright critique of the government's handling of the epidemic more generally, a dynamic which in itself demands an explanation that however falls outside this particular inquiry. This dynamic does nonetheless suggest that advocates for a stronger political response have to take into account a complex mix of political and personal considerations to successfully mobilise individuals in criticism of the government.

This conclusion is strengthened further by testing for a pattern on how "personal loss" correlates with three other political opinions and statements. Arguably, if it was the case that "personal loss" generated a more critical outlook on politics in general and the government in particular, this would be picked up by the three questions: do you disapprove of how President Thabo Mbeki has performed his job in the past 12 months; do you feel close to any particular political party; would you vote if there were elections for national government tomorrow? Table 26 shows the percentages of South Africans, those who have not and those who have experienced a personal loss respectively, who agree with the three statements.

We can see that the opinions held by those who have and those who have not experienced a personal loss to AIDS differ substantially only in five instances (highlighted in bold). The analysis does not prove that experiencing personal loss causes people to be more critical in these five instances, but indicates that this might be the case.

Table 26. Political opinions and personal loss, in percent of total

	Disapproves of President Mbeki's job performance over past twelve months		Does not feel close to any political party		Would not vote in election tomorrow	
	No loss	Loss	No loss	Loss	No loss	Loss
All South Africans	42.1	39.8	36.1	26.1	23.6	18.6
Black	32.3	38.1	24.5	25.2	15.5	18.6
Black male	30.5	31.9	20.5	20.8	10.6	16.7
Black female	34.4	43.1	29.8	28.6	22.0	20.3
Black urban	35.2	41.3	25.1	25.4	14.7	18.2
Black rural	29.5	34.5	23.9	24.5	16.3	19.1

Source: Afrobarometer survey South Africa 2002. The numbers indicate percentages of people who disapprove of President Mbeki's job performance over the last twelve months, who do not feel close to any political party, and who would not vote in the next election. A difference in percentage is noted as 'substantial' only if it exceeds the survey's 2.1 percentages margin of error.

Our conclusion on the basis of this statistical analyses is, on the one hand, that the epidemic has begun to shape a pattern in public opinion, a pattern in South Africans' opinions that does not feature across all of the Afrobarometer countries. A person's experience of personal loss is a moderately strong predictor of his/her preference for the government to prioritise development resources for the fight against the epidemic.

Given that the South African epidemic has entered a stage now when the number of AIDS-related deaths has started to rise sharply, we would expect this to generate a growing sentiment within the ANC's main support base for a stronger response against the epidemic, even at the cost of other development-related policy issues. However, the more direct and, for the government, potentially more difficult effect on people's political criticism of its performance is more limited. There were some indications in the 2002 Afrobarometer survey that there is a link between peoples' opinions on these two questions in the sense that people who want to prioritise more resources for AIDS are more likely also to be critical of the president's job performance during the past 12 months (Pearson's r = .103 at .01 level of significance). These indications are a warning signal to government and political parties that if the immediacy and effectiveness of the political response is not seen to correspond with people's harsh experiences of the epidemic, it has the potential to transform into a political issue that can shape electoral outcomes.

7.2 POLITICAL PARTICIPATION AND HIV/AIDS

A problematic hypothesis about the impact of the epidemic relates to levels of participation in the democratic process and in civil society activism in general, an effect that can either reduce or boost such participation. There are several examples of how, in South Africa, the fight against the epidemic by civil society organisations has built successfully on the legacies, strategies, networks and personalities that were active in the struggle against apartheid. These examples would suggest that the epidemic has re-mobilised civic activism in fighting for social justice in the form of medication against AIDS and the prevention and de-stigmatisation of HIV, with the activism of the Treatment Action Campaign (TAC) being the most notable example. Other indications suggest that people are de-mobilised by the epidemic, either because they have lost hope of an effective political response or because they are too busy providing home-based care for their own or someone else's AIDS-related illness or AIDS orphans to engage themselves politically. Of course, both these experiences exist and both simultaneously give shape to what is society's joint response to the epidemic. Our inquiry in this section will explore if either of these hypotheses can be traced in the Afrobarometer survey data.

As was mentioned in section 1.4, a survey instrument like the Afrobarometer cannot ask direct questions on the interviewees' HIV status or the status of those in their care since the stigma that is attached to the epidemic would severely undermine the validity of the responses. The Afrobarometer survey instead includes two sets of questions that will be used as proxies for the direct and indirect effects of the epidemic, the first relates to the home-based care a person provides for orphans, sick family members or her/his own illness, and the second relates to the person's physical and mental health. People were asked if they provide home-based care for orphans, for family or household members, or for their own illness, and if they do, for how many hours a day. We need to point out that these questions will of course also capture home-based care that is not related to AIDS, a fact that should be taken into account when the numbers are interpreted and analysed further. To allow for a more generalised and powerful test of the effect on participation by those who provide home-based care, we created a scale by collapsing the three questions on home-based care.[24] In the following we will therefore not be able to make a distinction between different recipients of such care; a distinction that in any case has little relevance in our discussion more broadly. Table 27 details how the levels of home-based care vary between the countries that were included in the Afrobarometer surveys. The numbers represent the mean value for the different countries, but we can give only a rough translation to what those values imply in terms of actual hours spent. The value .33 signifies that the average person spends less than one hour a day on home-based care (as in Namibia), while the highest possible value 4.0 would indicate that a person spends virtually all day providing all three kinds of home-based care. The different values in between .33 and 4.0 imply either that a person spends a lot of time providing one type of care, or that s/he spends some time providing two or three types of care. It is easiest to think of the numbers as relative indicators of the amount of time spent by people every day, with 0.0 meaning no time at all, and 4.0 meaning that the full day is spent providing home-based care.

Table 27. Average amount of home-based care per day per person

Botswana	1.57	Namibia	0.32	Zambia	1.97
Ghana	1.08	Nigeria	1.43	Cape Verde	1.19
Lesotho	2.02	South Africa	0.83	Kenya	1.22
Malawi	2.43	Tanzania	1.18	Mozambique	1.93
Mali	1.23	Uganda	2.17	Senegal	1.21

Source: Afrobarometer surveys 2002-2003. For interpretation, see text above.

We note that the South African mean value is the second lowest (after Namibia). On the basis of this information it would seem that the "average" South African is not particularly busy with home-based care when compared with the same average citizens in the southern African region. An additional form of presentation of this data that provides further information on a select group of countries indicates how the "time profiles" of home-based care varies in the different countries and among all of the 15 countries taken together (see figure 4 below). South Africa's profile is quite clear in that a very large minority (41.3 %) spend no time at all on home-based care and that the numbers of the people who do decreases as the amount of time increases. Uganda and Malawi, the two countries with the highest means, share a profile that is very different to South Africa's. In both these countries very few people spend no or little time on home-based care, with numbers increasing with an increase in time, and both countries have a considerable number of people carrying an extreme burden. The average profile for all the 15 countries in the survey is naturally more even across the different amounts of time spent.

Figure 4. The 'time profile' of home-based care in selected countries

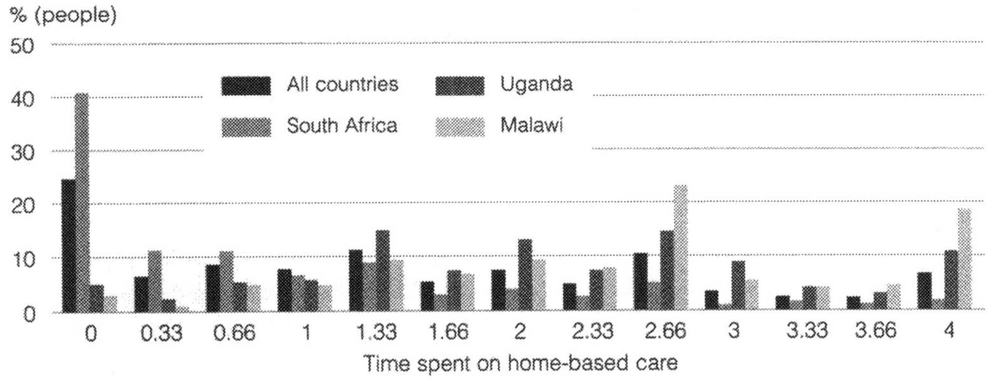

Source: Afrobarometer surveys 2002-2003. Calculations by authors.

There are a number of possible more general explanations for the differences between the countries. One would be the ability of the health care system in the countries to provide the necessary care so as to alleviate the burdens placed on private citizens. Another difference would be in what phase the epidemic was when the survey was conducted in 2002. One could make the argument that the relatively low numbers of people who provide home-based care in South Africa can be explained by both these factors; a better than average health care system and an epidemic that, in 2002, had only recently entered the phase when increasing numbers of people needed care due to AIDS-related illnesses. A third possible explanation for South Africa's "profile" could be the very heterogeneous character of South African society. However, when we isolated certain groups in the South African society who we know are more vulnerable to the direct or indirect effects of the epidemic, their respective profiles were only marginally different from that for all South Africans. In no instance did a South African profile match those of, for instance, Uganda and Malawi (see figure 5).

Figure 5. The 'time profile' of different groups of South Africans

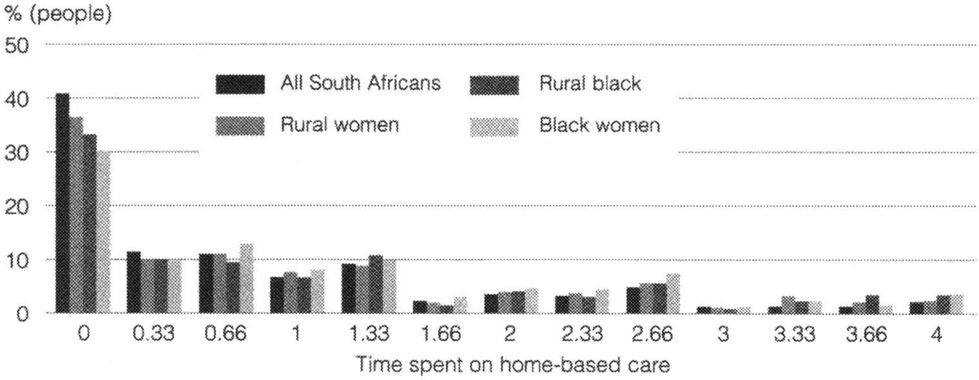

Source: Afrobarometer South African survey 2002. Calculations by authors.

The next step in our analysis, once we have described the quantity and "profile" of the amount of home-based care that people provide, is to test whether their responsibility for such care somehow affects their ability or willingness to be politically active in civil society, as well as to perform certain civic duties that are necessary for them to take part in elections. In a series of correlation analyses we tested whether the degree to which a person was providing home-based care was linked to her/his degree of activism in civil society (see table 28).[25] The hypothesis that providers of home-based care become inactive in civil society would be confirmed if these tests generate negative coefficients that are statistically significant – signifying that the more a person is busy with providing home-based care, the less active s/he is in civil society. The opposite hypothesis would be confirmed if positive coefficients are statistically significant, and the null-hypothesis, that providing home-based care is not a predictor of civil society activism at all, would be "confirmed" by weak coefficients that are not statistically significant. Before we comment on the results of these analyses we need to point out that they do not enable us to say anything about whether the burden of home-based care causes people to become more or less active in civil society. More complicated theoretical and statistical analyses could follow where either the first or second hypothesis has been confirmed, but we have no ambition to take the analyses that far in this present inquiry.

Table 28. Membership and activism in civil society, and home-based care

	Membership				Activity			
	Religious group	Trade union or farmers' org.	Professional or business org.	Community or developmet self-help org.	Discuss politics with friends	Attend community meeting	Got together with others to raise an issue	Attend demonstration or protest march
All	.075*	.022	-.024	.112**	-.041*	.192**	.121**	.049*
Black	.076**	.028	-.013	.074**	-.091**	.115**	.039	-.022
Black rural	.025	.046	-.015	.086*	-.084*	.116**	.075*	.001
Black women	.048	.027	-.040	.054	-.077*	.115**	.049	.010
Rural women	.008	-.007	-.038	.061	-.061	.198**	.130**	.041

Source: Afrobarometer survey South Africa 2002.Correlation coefficients (Pearson's r) between, on the one hand, different forms of membership and activity in civil society, and, on the other, the burden of providing home-based care. * indicates statistical significance on .05 level, and ** indicates statistical significance on .01 level.

The results indicate that the null-hypothesis dominates the picture since most coefficients are weak and not statistically significant; meaning that, in 2002, a person's responsibility for providing home-based care was a poor predictor of the degree to which s/he took an active part in civil society activism. There are however three notable general exceptions to that conclusion. Those who provide home-based care are somewhat more likely to be members of local development organisations and a great deal more likely to attend community meetings. On the other hand they are somewhat less likely to discuss politics with friends. One more detailed result is also worth commenting on. Many accounts identify rural women as particularly burdened by the responsibilities of providing home-based care, but we can see here that this experience is combined with a reasonably strong likelihood to meet with others with a common interest. The results might indicate that while rural women carry heavy responsibilities, they do so in a context of a relatively strong social capital that enables them to act collectively to try to make their plight a little easier. On the other hand, the "snapshot" image of civil society activism that the survey provides does not tell us anything about possible dynamic trends in these figures. It might very well be the case that the likelihood of this group of women to be active in civil society was even higher a few years prior to the survey in 2002.

A related set of hypotheses predicts what home-based care implies for a person's willingness or ability to perform the civic duties necessary to vote – to obtain the relevant ID document and to register to vote. As was the case above, either a person's motivation to perform these "duties" is reduced by the despair and frustrations caused by having to provide home-based care, or these hardships generate an awareness and mobilise a determination to ensure that as many votes as possible are cast in favour of a political programme that people hope will assist them in their harsh situation. The null-hypothesis, as above, would indicate that home-based care has little or no impact on people's willingness or ability to perform these critical civic duties. A related variable has been included to test if the burdens of home-based care impacts on people's level of general satisfaction with the South African democracy.[26]

The results indicate clearly that, in 2002, the responsibility for providing home-based care did not interfere with people's ability or undermine their willingness to perform these critical civic duties. If anything, a few significant positive coefficients would suggest that people with responsibility for home-based care are more likely to take a responsibility to ensure their active participation in the electoral process. The test against people's satisfaction

Table 29. Does providing home-based care affect civic duties and opinion on SA's democracy?

	Easy to obtain ID document	Easy to register to vote	Satisfaction with democracy
All	.071*	.061*	.028
Black	.039	.024	.005
Black rural	.086*	.065	-.027
Black women	.047	.065	-.020
Rural women	.044	.111*	-.070

Source: Afrobarometer survey South Africa 2002.Correlation coefficients (Pearson's r) between, on the one hand, two different civic duties and an opinion about democracy, and, on the other, the burden of providing home-based care. * indicates statistical significance on .05 level, and ** indicates statistical significance on .01 level.

with the South African democracy shows that, in 2002, the many frustrations and hardships of home-based care did not generate a general dissatisfaction with the South African democracy; home-based care was not at all a predictor for people's views in that regard.

Conclusions

In concluding this section of our analysis we note that although increasing numbers of people are directly or indirectly affected by the epidemic, there has yet to emerge a clear indication in the survey data of a political reaction as a consequence of this. Where we can see such a clear effect it merely suggests that people who have experienced a personal loss to AIDS would like the government to prioritise its spending so as to avoid further losses. The same traumatic experience does not lead to criticism of the government more generally nor of the president more specifically who in 2002 personified the government's response to the epidemic. Further, the Afrobarometer information from 2002 provides no basis for the general argument that people who are busy providing home-based care in one form or another are more likely to be inactive in civil society or not take the personal responsibility to ensure they are able to take full part in the electoral process. If anything, the stronger indication points in the opposite direction. While these concluding comments, arguably, are valid on the basis of our analysis of the data, it is important also to point out the limits of these conclusions.

The first such limit is that the information is somewhat dated. Research on survey data often seek to test general theoretical hypotheses of a kind that does not require current data. But this is not the case with analyses of the impacts of the HIV/AIDS epidemic on the democracies in South and southern Africa. An epidemic does not, by definition, cause a constant level of impact on a society. Since it spreads rapidly in the population, its effect also increases rapidly, albeit with a time lag in relation to its incidence in that population. In the context of AIDS in southern Africa, two years is a long time in which the effects of the epidemic rise sharply. This means that the impact we have noted in South Africa above on the basis of data from 2002 is not necessarily accurate for what impact the epidemic has at present. A further limitation is that a single survey is a "snapshot" of reality that does not tell us anything about trends in the impact we are analysing. Since the questions we have worked with in this section were not included in the first round of Afrobarometer surveys in 2000, it is only when we can work on the data from the third round of surveys, planned for 2004-2005, that we can comment on the direction of any such trends. Taken together, these drawbacks with the data should caution the reader to remember that the epidemic is not only a "moving target", but it is also a target with an impact that grows constantly both in extent and severity.

The fact that most of the tests in relation to non-registration were confirmed indicates some support for the argument that the higher the impact of HIV prevalence in a province, the more likely it is that those in the more vulnerable ages do not bother to register to vote. If this held true, it signals a worrying tendency of alienation from the democratic process by the women, who arguably need it the most.

Chapter 8

Exploring the Impact on Levels of Registration and Voter Turnout

8.1 INTRODUCTION

The electoral statistics for the 2004 elections set a downward trend in voter participation. Despite the fact that increasing numbers of South Africans have the right to vote and more of them registered to take part in the democratic process than in the two previous elections, fewer of them actually turned out to vote, either by choice or by circumstance. This observation relates to one of the most central questions for social science research: why would a person spend limited resources to participate in a collective action from which s/he stands to gain, but that would suffer only very marginally if s/he abstained. This general problem of collective action applies very well to research on voter participation in democratic elections. In pure rational and "economic" terms, a selfish calculation by the individual voter would have him/her stay at home while everyone else makes the effort to vote. The risk, of course, is that everyone else makes that same calculation with the result that the democratic process derails completely, despite being preferred by everyone. For the sake of democracy it is therefore a very good thing that most people see beyond this selfish calculation and spend some resources on sharing the responsibility for sustaining their democratic system of government.

Scholars are working with different hypotheses to try to understand what causes the differences in participation across different countries and different categories of voters (Norris 2002). On a global scale, factors such as level of development and institutional differences (ie mainly the electoral system and processes of registration) play a part in the explanation, and within countries many focus on how the youth appear to prefer other means of more direct political participation.

These hypotheses share the basic assumption that the potential voter can take part in the election, but that s/he for one or other reason does not want to. What has been suggested in the literature is that the HIV/AIDS epidemic introduces a new hypothesis with the reverse logic: that the voter wants to take full part in the election but that s/he cannot. The main purpose of our analysis in this chapter is to put this hypothesis to the test in the context of the 2004 elections in South Africa.

Table 30 provides the numbers on the national level for the three South African national and provincial elections and thus details our initial comments that in 2004 there were more people with the right to vote than previously, and

Table 30. Voter participation in South Africa's three national elections

Year	Voting Age Population (VAP)	Registered voters	Total votes	Vote/Reg. (%)	Vote/VAP (%)	Reg/VAP (%)
1994	22 709 152	—	19 533 498	—	86.0	—
1999	22 589 369	18 172 751	16 228 462	89.3	71.8	80.4
2004	A 27 865 537	B 20 674 926	B 15 863 554	76.7	56.9	74.2

Source: Figures from Independent Electoral Commission for the 1994 and 1999 elections as reported in Reynolds, 1994 and 1999b respectively. A Statistics SA (2004) mid-2004 estimates, see endnote for further details.
B Independent Electoral Commission (total votes includes spoilt ballot papers).

more of them were registered to vote, but fewer than in the two previous elections actually turned out to vote.

The obviously strange feature of the numbers in table 30 is the very high increase in the voting-age-population (VAP) – that is, South African citizens 18 years old or older[27] – between the 1999 and 2004 elections. Such anomalies would perhaps explain the apparent mistrust among scholars of official demographic statistics. One commentator on the election result chose therefore to disregard the VAP altogether in his comment and only discuss the ratio between registered and actual voters (Sachs, 2004). While this strategy might become necessary where the demographic statistics are wholly missing or completely unreliable, this is arguably not the case in South Africa. We would caution the reader not to diminish the analysis by completely denying the information that those statistics hold. One could even make the argument, as Philippa Norris does in her authoritative analysis of voter participation, that it is imperative for the researcher to always include the VAP in the analysis so as not to hide the disenfranchisement of an otherwise "invincible" section of the population (Norris, 2004:40). This advice is particularly relevant for our inquiry as we are testing the hypothesis that the direct or indirect effects of HIV/AIDS might reduce people's ability and/or willingness to register and vote in the election.

It was for these reasons that it was very timely for our research that Statistics SA, the authority tasked with providing official statistics in South Africa, published its 2004 mid-year estimate of the South African population at the end of July, only a few months after the elections. Since the population estimates in the report also include residents who are not citizens – and therefore do not have the vote – demographers at Statistics SA suggested we should generate the VAP that was current for the 2004 elections by multiplying the numbers by the factor .9851817, which was the percent of residents in South Africa in the 2001 Census who were South African citizens. This calculation was done on the estimates provided by Statistics SA to generate the percentages of electoral participation for the different age cohorts and provinces that we present below in table 31.

Table 31. Electoral participation across provinces and gender, 2004

	Reg./VAP			Vote/Reg.	Vote/VAP
	male	female	total	total	total
Western Cape	70.4	78.8	74.7	71.3	53.2
Eastern Cape	66.9	77.1	72.5	79.3	57.5
Northern Cape	74.3	80.7	77.5	74.7	57.9
Free State	68.8	75.9	72.5	77.8	56.4
KwaZulu-Natal	63.4	73.7	68.9	72.8	50.2
North West	69.6	80.8	75.1	75.6	56.7
Gauteng	73.2	80.3	76.6	74.2	56.9
Mpumalanga	74.4	81.6	78.1	78.3	61.2
Limpopo	65.3	90.4	78.5	74.8	58.7
National	**68.9**	**79.2**	**74.2**	**76.7**	**56.9**

Source: Statistics SA (2004) and the Independent Electoral Commission.

We can note considerable differences between provincial figures and the national average, in one instance of more than six percentages in the most problematic case of the "vote/VAP" ratio in the KwaZulu-Natal province.

The ratio between registered voters and VAP can be broken down further by looking at different age cohorts by province. As we focus on the younger voters the ratio drops from 74.2% for the whole electorate, to 69.2% for those between 18 and 49, to a very low 52.1% for first-time voters. It is important to note the wide differences among these youngest voters between the sexes, but even more so between the provinces.

Table 32. Ratio between registered voters and VAP, by age cohort, sex and province

	Registered voters as percent of VAP for different age cohorts								
	18 years and older			18 to 49 years			18 to 22 years		
	male	female	total	male	female	total	male	female	total
Western Cape	70.4	78.8	74.7	66.3	74.4	70.4	52.6	59.7	56.2
Eastern Cape	66.9	77.1	72.5	61.1	70.7	66.2	40.2	46.8	43.5
Northern Cape	74.3	80.7	77.5	71.7	77.8	74.7	57.3	62.7	59.9
Free State	68.8	75.9	72.5	65.8	70.9	68.4	48.7	53.9	51.3
KwaZulu-Natal	63.4	73.7	68.9	59.2	67.3	63.4	42.7	48.0	45.3
North West	69.6	80.8	75.1	65.9	75.5	70.5	53.2	59.4	56.2
Gauteng	73.2	80.3	76.6	69.8	76.2	72.8	64.3	66.0	65.2
Mpumalanga	74.4	81.6	78.1	70.8	76.3	73.6	51.9	57.4	54.7
Limpopo	65.3	90.4	78.5	61.0	79.9	70.8	43.3	54.1	48.7
National	**68.9**	**79.2**	**74.2**	**64.9**	**73.4**	**69.2**	**49.2**	**55.0**	**52.1**

Source: The Independent Electoral Commission. Calculations by authors.

Finally, a particularly interesting feature of the report by Statistics SA is that it details its estimate of the South African population in an "actual" estimate as well as in a "counterfactual" estimate that presents what the population estimate should have been if the HIV/AIDS epidemic had not reduced the population. The report presents its estimates for the South African population in mid-2004 in age cohorts of five years (0-4, 5-9, 10-14, etc.) and by the four racial groups. If we calculate the VAP on both sets of statistics we will be able to identify the extent to which, according to these estimates, the epidemic has reduced the VAP for the South African elections in 2004. Given that the age 18 falls within one of the age cohorts we have had to work with the assumption that the estimated numbers within the cohort 15-19 are distributed equally across the five years and then multiply this number by two, according to the formula (estimate / 5) x 2. As could be expected, our calculations generate the greatest reduction in VAP within the age cohort 18-49 years that is most severely affected by the epidemic (see table 33.) We can note also that the differences in prevalence between the racial groups, as well as between men and women are reflected in these statistics.

Our analysis so far has sought to generate the relevant information from the electoral and demographic data and comment on the differences between the sexes, different age cohorts and the provinces. We shall now see if these differences can be said to confirm the general hypothesis that the HIV/AIDS epidemic caused a reduction in the level of participation in the 2004 elections. Our

Table 33. Estimated reduction of VAP due to AIDS

	18-29 years		18-49 years		18 years and older	
	estimate	%	estimate	%	estimate	%
Black	236 643	2.6	968 057	5.3	1 088 582	4.9
Male	68 089	1.5	466 325	5.1	552 450	5.1
Female	168 554	3.7	501 732	5.5	536 132	4.7
Coloured	8 740	1.0	42 795	2.0	48 279	1.8
Male	2 363	0.5	20 399	2.0	24 232	1.9
Female	6 377	1.4	22 396	2.1	24 047	1.8
Asian	907	0.4	4 370	0.8	5 213	0.7
Male	236	0.2	2 068	0.7	2 660	0.7
Female	671	0.5	2 302	0.8	2 553	0.6
White	6 845	1.0	41 500	2.0	51 947	1.5
Male	1 634	0.5	19 552	1.9	26 618	1.6
Female	5 211	1.5	21 948	2.1	25 329	1.5
SA Total	**181 135**	**2.3**	**1 056 723**	**4.6**	**1 194 082**	**4.1**
Male	**72 323**	**1.3**	**508 344**	**4.5**	**606 021**	**4.3**
Female	**180 812**	**3.3**	**548 379**	**4.7**	**588 061**	**3.9**

Source: Statistics SA (2004). Numbers calculated by authors. 'Estimate' refers to the difference between the estimates in the 'no AIDS' and 'AIDS' scenarios, which is then given as the percentage of the total of that age cohort.

statistical tests in the section below will not be able to prove any such causal link, but they might generate the basis for the argument that the two are linked.

8.2 FORMULATING AND CONTEXTUALISING THE HYPOTHESES

The following three general hypotheses will guide our statistical tests for correlation between electoral and epidemiological data:

- People who are HIV positive choose to not participate in elections since they are frustrated and disillusioned by a weak political response from the formal political system;
- People who are sick with AIDS-related illnesses cannot participate in the electoral process because of the effort participation implies, particularly in terms of various possible bureaucratic processes, transport to the polling station and standing in line to vote;
- People who provide home-based care for AIDS orphans, or for family or friends who are AIDS sick, or who take care of their own AIDS-related illness, either choose to not participate for the same reason as in (1) above or they are simply too busy to spend their very limited resources participating in elections.

To test these hypotheses we shall relate some of the electoral data above to the provincial percentages of HIV estimates by the Department of Health, and the projections of the percentage of people who are ill with AIDS, by province, from the Actuarial Society of South Africa (ASSA) model. Before we proceed with the tests, however, we need to recall the finding by Olive Shisana (2002) and her team in the Human Sciences Research Council (HSRC) household survey that as many as 75% of infected South Africans were not aware of being infected, a circumstance that considerably reduces the possible effect of the first hypothesis since we cannot in any way assume that estimated infection rates will be reflected automatically in levels of non-participation as the hypothesis suggests. The hypothesis is still relevant, but it has a considerably weaker effect on participation than we first assumed.

In a similar fashion our expectations of the effect on participation by hypotheses two and three must be downscaled on the basis of the information we gained from the Afrobarometer survey, as discussed above in chapter seven. The proxy questions for HIV/AIDS, as well as the precise questions for providing home-based care, had little if any effect on whether people thought it was easy or difficult to obtain an ID document and to register to vote.

When these Afrobarometer findings are taken together, and with the addition of the finding from the HSRC, we can conclude that existing data suggests that we will not find a strong effect on electoral participation from the direct or indirect consequences of the epidemic. We present our results in a summary form in table 34 on the opposite page. The reader should further note that the analysis is done on the level of provinces (N=9), which has the implication for the statistical analysis that was discussed in section 1.4.

We can see that three of the four hypotheses regarding non-registration by eligible voters were confirmed, but that the result was somewhat more diverse for the hypotheses about non-voting by registered voters.

Two of the results deserve to be highlighted somewhat. The fact that most of the tests in relation to non-registration were confirmed indicates some support for the argument that the higher the impact of HIV prevalence in a province, the more likely it is that those in the more vulnerable ages (18-49 years) do not bother to register to vote. If this holds to be true, it signals a worrying tendency of alienation from the democratic process by the women, who arguably need it the most. We shall return to this finding and explore it further through another methodology, focus group discussions, in chapter ten. Secondly, the fact that hypothesis three was confirmed, albeit not very strongly, in relation to non-voting by registered voters suggests that there is a more general relevance to the complaints about the delivery of the special vote that we noted above, and that this insufficiency did disenfranchise people who were sick with AIDS. As we noted in chapter five the Independent Electoral Commission (IEC) does not seem to have the data available on the details of the applications and delivery of special votes that would be necessary to explore further the solidity of this statistical finding. Our results here can perhaps serve as an additional indication that more needs to be done for the special vote to become as effective as possible to make sure that those who are ill with AIDS, or any other disease, actually get the chance to vote.

Table 34. Tests of hypotheses about impact of HIV/AIDS on participation in 2004 election, (N=9)

Observations	Non-registration by eligible voters	Non-voting by registered voters
Hypotheses	(1) Voters who are directly or indirectly affected by HIV/AIDS are disillusioned by the political response to AIDS or exhausted by the burdens they carry withdraw completely from participation rather than vote for another party. (2) The dynamic of (1) should apply even more to adult women (15-49 years) who have higher prevalence levels than men. (3) In the case of young women, who we know are particularly affected by the virus, the effect of disillusionment is increased further (4) AIDS sick voters fail to re-register as they move to live with extended family to get 'home-based' care.	(1) HIV-positive voters are disillusioned by government policy on HIV/AIDS; they withdraw completely rather than vote for another party. (2) AIDS sick voters are too ill to make it to the voting station. (3) The special vote was not effective in assisting those sick with AIDS. (4) The voters' roll is inaccurate due to unrecorded AIDS-related deaths.
Expectations	(1) Positive correlation between levels of non-registration and estimates of HIV prevalence. (2) A stronger positive correlation than in (1). (3) A considerable positive correlation between levels of non-registration among young women and estimates of HIV prevalence among young women. (4) Positive correlation between levels of non-registration and projections of numbers of AIDS-sick.	(1) Positive correlation between levels of non-voting and estimates of HIV prevalence. (2) Positive correlation between levels of non-voting and projections of numbers of AIDS-sick. (3) Negative correlation between number of special votes as percentage of total vote and projections of numbers of AIDS-sick. (4) Positive correlation between levels of non-voting and projections of numbers of AIDS deaths since the census in 2001 (i.e. projected numbers of AIDS deaths between the years 2001 and 2004).
Findings	(1) Confirmed. *Pearson's r* = .504 (2) Confirmed: *Pearson's r* = .590 (3) Rejected. *Pearson's r* = .346 (4) Confirmed. *Pearson's r* = .344	(1) Rejected for all provinces (*Pearson's r* = -.370),. (2) Rejected for all provinces (*Pearson's r* = .368) (3) Confirmed when outlier province WC was excluded (*Pearson's r* = -.142) but rejected when WC was included (*Pearson's r* = .248).28 (4) Rejected for all provinces (*Pearson's r* = -.267), but confirmed when outlier province WC was excluded (*Pearson's r* = ..102).

Source: Electoral data from the IEC, epidemiological data from DoH and ASSA model as detailed previously in this report. Calculations by authors.

CONCLUSION

Our analysis in this chapter generated additional information on the VAP in the 2004 South African election. This is not to deny that the numbers we present are ambiguous due to uncertainties about the reliability of the basic demographic data, the 2001 Census. We argued however that the VAP is an important part of any analysis of electoral participation, especially when the focus of the analysis is the risk of systematic non-participation by one or more groups in the population. Our tests of the hypotheses to explain the variations in participation indicated that there is a link to be explored further between non-participation and the HIV/AIDS epidemic, which is what we intend to do in the next two chapters.

Whereas KwaZulu-Natal in 2003 had the highest mortality in absolute numbers among women voters aged 30-39 years with 11 065 deaths and the Free State recorded the highest number of deaths in relative numbers for the same year for women of 30-49 years, the rate at which mortality in relative numbers increased between 1999 and 2003 was highest in Limpopo and Mpumalanga.

CHAPTER 9

ANALYSING LEVELS AND PROFILES OF MORTALITY ON THE SOUTH AFRICAN VOTERS' ROLL

> *"...Unless one is completely insensitive, one can't but help notice the ages of those who have died. Just look at the first two numbers of the person's ID and it will tell you the year they were born in. When you delete an entry for someone with an ID starting 15 or 25, one can be philosophical and say they have had a good innings. But when one deletes IDs starting with the numbers 84 or even 74, then one realises that these South Africans died in their 20s and 30s..." GDA Pullman, letter to the Natal Witness on purging dead voters from the voter's roll.*

9.1 INTRODUCTION

Up to this point in our report we have used electoral data from the Independent Electoral Commission (IEC) to detail levels of registration and turnout in the 2004 election and we have consulted various estimates of HIV prevalence and projections of AIDS-related mortality to detail the effects of the epidemic. In this chapter we shall attempt to merge electoral and epidemiological data in an analysis of the impact of the HIV/AIDS epidemic on the electoral process in South Africa that is based on a unique set of data that was provided to us by the IEC.

Our initial requests for information from the IEC were in part motivated by the general concern in the literature that if sharp increases in mortality due to AIDS are not correctly accounted for on the voters' roll this opens a margin for manipulation and cheating that undermines the legitimacy of the whole election. The IEC was soon able to put our concerns in this regard to rest as they convinced us of the efficiency and accuracy of the process with which they remove dead voters from the roll (see chapter five). It is the IEC's proficiency with this information that, after a second round of enquiries from us, resulted in a set of information that has never been compiled in this fashion.

On the basis of this information we shall present an analysis in the form of graphs, maps and tables on the basis of which we make the argument that the epidemic has indeed made its mark on the South African electorate in a way that should further strengthen the political resolve to address the epidemic with a sense of urgency. What emerges from our analysis, arguably, is the veritable "smoking gun" of AIDS-related mortality among the South African electorate. The analysis and the information we can present here therefore does not only speak to our more specific purpose in this report – to explore what impact HIV/AIDS might have had on the 2004 elections – but also addresses the more general question of whether mortality from AIDS is as problematic as is argued by many analysts and activists who work in the field. This debate need not be reduced to one between "mainstream" and "dissident" views on the epidemic – that is, whether HIV causes AIDS or not – but is one between those who argue that current estimates of HIV prevalence and AIDS mortality are correct (given a level of inherent uncertainty) and those who argue that such estimates are considerably overstated.

One of the most prominent and effective communicators of the latter argument, journalist and author Rian Malan, argued recently in the *Sunday Times* (3 October 2004) that AIDS experts exaggerate the devastation brought by the epidemic. At the core of Malan's argument is a deep mistrust of the experts who generate the estimates. In Malan's analysis these experts, with most journalists in an uncritical media, represent an AIDS establishment that lives comfortably off the funding it is given on the basis of its own alarmist information about the epidemic. The information we can present in this chapter is particularly powerful in the context of these somewhat inflamed debates since it comprises data that has not been generated through complex statistical estimates or projections based on problematic assumptions. Our information details mortality among the South African electorate as it is reflected directly on the South African voters' roll via the Population Register; every number represents an actual deceased person. Our analysis below will show that South African voters are indeed dying in numbers and according to an age profile that, arguably, defies any other explanation than AIDS. While critics are free to question our motivations for presenting this information and challenge our analysis, we expect that all will trust the validity and reliability of the information.[29]

9.1.1 THE DATA FROM THE SOUTH AFRICAN VOTERS' ROLL

The data set contains the following information:

- The number of registered voters at the end of the years 1999, 2000, 2001, 2002 and 2003;
- The total number of deceased registered voters for the years 1999, 2000, 2001, 2002 and 2003, per gender and per age cohort (18-19; 20-29; 30-39: 40-49; 50-59; 60-69; 70-79; 80+);
- The number of registered voters at the end of the years 1999, 2000, 2001, 2002 and 2003, per gender, per age cohort (as above), per province and per municipality, and
- The total number of deceased registered voters for the years 1999, 2000, 2001, 2002 and 2003, per gender, per age cohort (as above), per province and per municipality.

This information is highly relevant for a number of analytical purposes. Demographers can use it to check the validity of the assumptions about mortality that they use in their models for estimation and political scientists will learn much about how levels of electoral registration vary between ages and gender and municipalities across the country. If the information is used in combination with other sources of data the number of possible usages is multiplied and only limited by the availability of such information at the relevant level of analysis.

Our usage and presentation of this information is in some aspects explorative.

By this we mean that since we are not qualified in demographic analysis we cannot authoritatively address the full complexities and implications of the data. It is clear to us that the data from the voters' roll cannot be assumed to be representative of all South African residents of the age 18 and older. Our analyses and comments are therefore not intended to imply such representivity. We leave it to qualified demographers to take the analysis further in this regard. This is however no real limitation of our research project. Given the overall theme of the report we are really interested only in analysing the implications of the epidemic for the South African electorate, the part of the population who at some stage were registered on the voters' roll. In other aspects our analysis of this information is argumentative in the sense that it is based on an argument of how the trends that emerge through our analysis should be interpreted. We base our argument on authoritative research and we seek to strengthen it further by establishing how it is linked to other sets of data.

9.1.2 CAVEATS, ARGUMENT AND METHODOLOGY

We realise that the analysis we will present below might be considered controversial and contestable on some grounds. In this section we will therefore try to be very clear and explicit about what factors and circumstances have to be considered when interpreting the data by presenting three such caveats:

- The data do not contain any information at all on the causes of death. It is therefore impossible to say with certainty how many of the deceased registered voters died from an AIDS-related disease;
- An increase in levels of mortality from one year to another – measured as a ratio between deceased and registered voters in the respective years (see below) – might to some extent be explained by an increased efficiency in the reporting and accounting of deaths by the relevant authorities, primarily the Department of Home Affairs;
- The information does not detail the total level of mortality in South Africa, but only the reported deaths of citizens who were registered to vote. Therefore, any analytical inferences made on the basis of the data exclude population groups such as citizens who are below the age of 18, adult citizens who had not registered to vote and non-citizens who reside in South Africa.

While our analysis will consider these caveats, they will not hinder us from making the argument that AIDS is the main cause behind the problematic "mortality profiles" that our analysis generates. This interpretation is based on the research we review briefly in section 9.1.3 below.

The basis for this argument is not immediately self-evident in the data set but we have to make some basic mathematical calculations to clarify the trend that sustains the argument. Even at first glance the absolute numbers in the data set appear to indicate that we are looking at an abnormal distribution of deaths among registered voters. By absolute numbers we mean the actual number of deaths as they are recorded by the IEC in the data set. But since an increase in absolute numbers might in part be explained by a corresponding increase in the number of registered voters, it is the relative number of deaths that is most relevant to our analysis here. By relative number we mean the number of deaths in a year as a percentage of the total number of registered voters during that year. Once we have established the relative number of deaths we will go one step further and work out the increase in the relative number of deaths between 1999 and 2003. This increase is calculated according to the following formula:

$$\frac{(\%\ \text{Deaths 2003} - \%\ \text{Deaths 1999})}{\%\ \text{Deaths 1999}} = \begin{array}{c}\%\ \text{Deaths 1999 in}\\ \text{relative number of}\\ \text{deaths from}\\ \text{1999 to 2003}\end{array}$$

% Deaths imply the relative number of deaths as explained above

By doing this simple calculation we make our analysis more precise since we can establish variations in the dynamic trend of how many voters died out of a defined number of registered voters.

9.1.3 RESEARCH ON HIV/AIDS AND MORTALITY IN SOUTH AFRICA

There are, to the best of our knowledge, two research publications that are particularly relevant as points of comparison with our data from the voters' roll. In 2001 Rob Dorrington et al published an extensive report – *The impact of HIV/AIDS on adult mortality in South Africa* – that was based on death statistics from the Department of Home Affairs' Population Register. This information was processed through the ASSA model to generate estimates of AIDS-related mortality among different ages and racial population groups as well as between men and women for South Africa and the nine provinces (Dorrington 2001). The result that the researchers emphasise is how mortality had increased sharply among young adults, and among young women in particular, peaking around 30-35 years. In his foreword to the report, the then-President of the Medical Research Council, Malegepuru Makgoba, also highlighted the fact that:

> *the pattern of mortality from natural causes in South Africa has shifted from the old to the young over the last decade particularly for young women – this is a unique phenomenon in biology (Dorrington 2001: 4).*

In a brief update of this analysis Bradshaw et al analyses the trends in the actual number of deaths as reported in the Population Register between 1998 and 2003. The increase in mortality among women is highlighted also in this report:

> *In the case of women 20-49 years, there has been an increase of 190% in the deaths registered which corresponds to a real increase in mortality of more than 150% once population growth and possible improvement in registration are taken into account (Bradshaw 2004: 3).*

Professor Bradshaw then concludes by saying:

> *The uncertainty about the precise number of AIDS deaths should not allow people to dismiss the impact of HIV/AIDS on mortality. There has been a massive rise in the total number of adult deaths in the last 6 years. Given the ages at which these additional deaths occurred and the change in the cause of death profile, they can largely be attributed to HIV/AIDS (2004: 4).*

Since our analysis of the data from the IEC will display the same general profiles and tendencies as the data and analyses presented by professors Dorrington and Bradshaw, we will argue that our information to a large extent corroborates the findings by South Africa's foremost analysts in the field.

9.2 GENERAL TRENDS IN THE DATA

We shall begin this section by clarifying some national trends in the data that are clear causes for concern as they, arguably, corroborate the hypotheses that AIDS mortality is impacting on the level and distribution of mortality among the South African electorate. In a second section we shall expand the analysis by clarifying how these trends vary between the different South African provinces and municipalities.

9.2.1 NATIONAL TRENDS

Between November 1998 and the end of 2003 a total of 1 488 242 – or roughly 1.5 million – voters were removed from the voters' roll due to death. From 1999 to 2003 the absolute number of deaths among the total South African electorate increased by 66% (from 215 583 in 1999 to 358 486 in 2003). The number of deceased voters per year is detailed in figure 6 in absolute as well as relative numbers.

Figure 6. Absolute and relative numbers of deceased voters per year

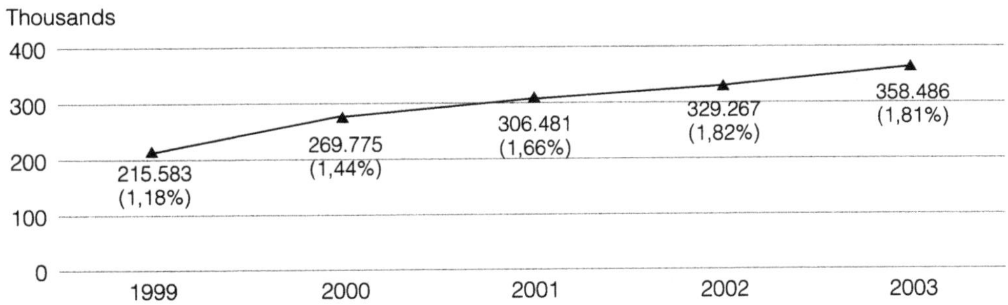

Source: IEC, 2004e. Calculations by authors.

The graph reveals that voters also died at an increasing rate in relative numbers. However, before we explore the relative numbers further, much important information is still hidden from us in the absolute numbers of death since we are here looking at an aggregate number for all registered voters. As we distinguish between the eight different age cohorts in figure 7 we shall see, as could be expected, that voters of different ages contribute differently to the increase in mortality.

Figure 7. Number of deceased voters by age group and year

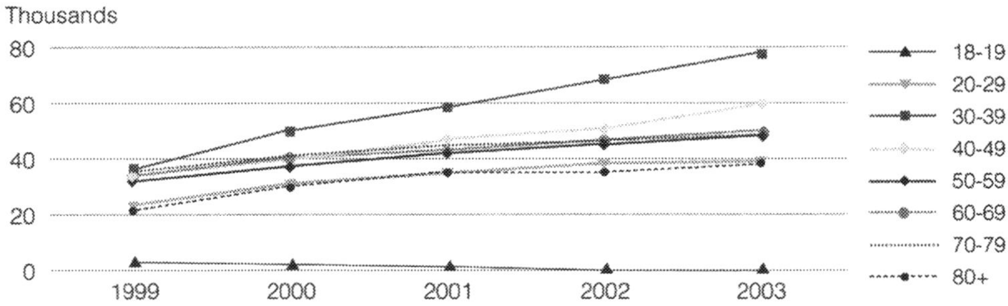

Source: IEC, 2000e. Calculations by authors.

We can see that mortality within the two age cohorts 30-39 and 40-49 year olds appears to increase at a higher rate than the other age cohorts. This would seem to correspond with the general expectation among demographers working on the epidemic that it is within this age span that AIDS mortality becomes most clearly visible. A different way of clarifying the extent to which the increase in mortality is concentrated to some age cohorts more than others is to calculate the percentages of which the different age cohorts contribute to the overall increase in mortality. Figure 8 clarifies, for instance, and most alarmingly, that the increase in mortality within the age cohort 30-39 years account for 29% of the total increase in morality among registered voters.

Figure 8. Percentage share of increase in mortality 1999=2003, by age group

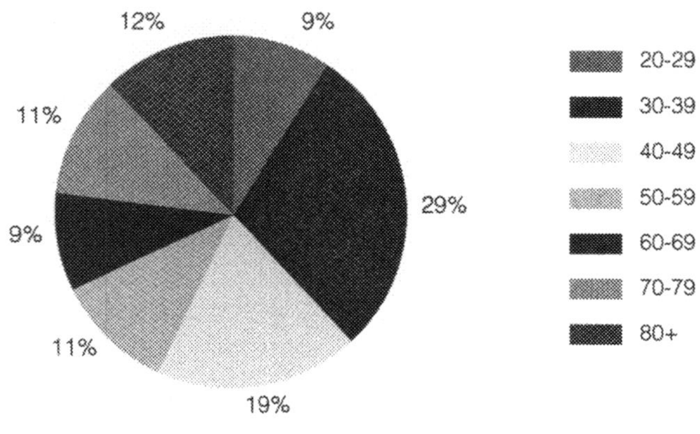

Source: IEC, 2004e. Calculations by authors.

The next distinction we shall explore is that between men and women. We start by presenting the mortality profiles for women and men separately. In figures 9 and 10 we will compare absolute numbers of deceased men and women in age cohorts 20 years and older for the years 1999 and 2003. But each graph also compares these profiles on the basis of two data sets. Our information from the voters' roll is here compared with the profiles that Professor Debbie Bradshaw and her colleagues generated on the basis of the Population Register (2004). We should note, however, that since we did not have access to the precise numbers of deaths in the data from the Population Register we worked out the numbers of deaths from the graphs as they are presented in the publication by Professor Bradshaw as precisely as we could. Even though this introduces some amount of imprecision in our reference to the data from the Population Register, the comparison will nevertheless provide a valuable test as to how, if at all, the mortality profile of the South African electorate differs substantially from that of the population in general. As we can see in the graphs below, the similarities between the two sets of data are very clear indeed. Since more people are registered in the Population Register than on the voters' roll, it would be expected that the lines for the Population Register indicate a higher number of deaths for the two years respectively, and that it does so for both women and men. The similarity we wish to emphasise here is that the particularly sharp increase in mortality for some age cohorts in the IEC data that we noted above is almost identically reflected in the data from the Population Register.

Figure 9. Comparing mortality profiles 1999 and 2003, women per age cohort

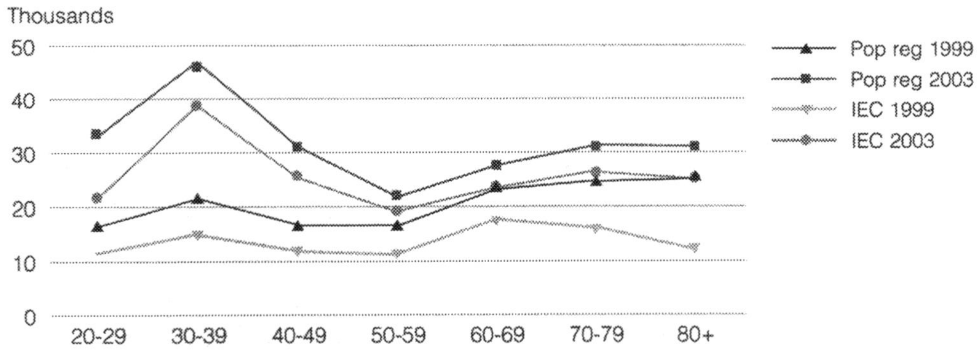

Source: IEC, 2004e and Bradshaw *et al*, 2004. Calculations by authors.

Figure 10. Comparing mortality profiles 1999 and 2003, men per age cohort

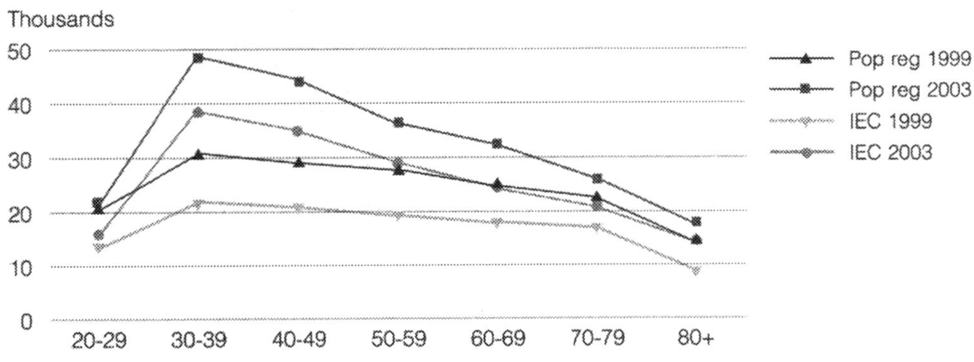

Source: IEC, 2000e and Bradshaw *et al*, 2004. Calculations by authors.

According to predictions of AIDS mortality we would expect women to die at a higher rate than men since they are more vulnerable to the virus in the first instance. However, the normal demographic "pattern" of mortality for South Africa is that higher numbers of men die at a younger age than do women; women have a higher average age than men. This pattern is found also in our data from the voters' roll, but only for the year 1999. In this year more men than women died in the six younger age cohorts and mortality among women surpasses that among men only in the age cohort 70-79 years as would be expected. But, as figure 11 details below, in 2000 this pattern shifted quite dramatically with mortality among 20-29-year-old women being higher than that among men. The figure also reveals that the major thrust of the increase we noted above in the age cohort 30-39 is caused by a sharp increase in mortality among women, an increase in which mortality among women surpassed that of men in 2003.

Figure 11. Number of deceased voters 20-29 and 30-39 years, per gender

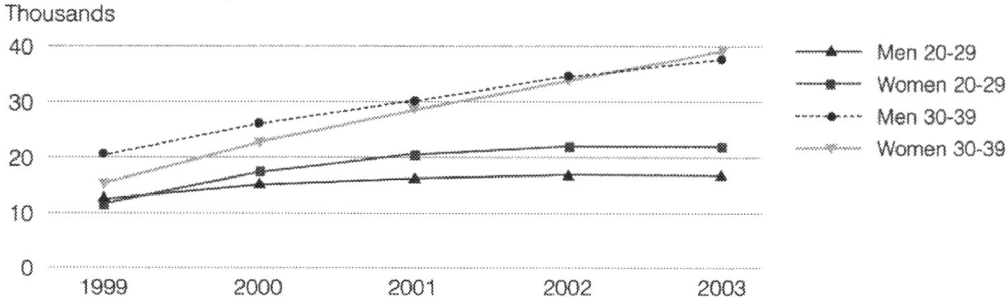

Source: IEC, 2000e. Calculations by authors.

Yet another way of analysing trends in the mortality statistics is to investigate what share, or what ratio, mortality in one group represents compared with another group, measured in absolute numbers of death. In a "healthy" population mortality among the younger sections of the population should, quite naturally, be lower compared with that of the older section of the population, ie showing a ratio much below 1. The South African mortality statistics, however, display a worrying trend in this regard. In their report from 2001 Dorrington et al show that the ratio of mortality between those who were 15-49 years old and those who were 50 years and older was increasing steadily between the years 1990 to 1999/2000. In 1990 this ratio was 0.31 for women and 0.66 for men, but ten years later it had increased to 0.78 for women and 1.00 for men. That is, in 1999-2000 mortality among young women (15-49 years old) was still lower than for women aged 50 and over, but the difference was considerably less compared with ten years earlier. For men, however, mortality among men below 50 years in 1999-2000 was equal to that of men 50 years and older. In table 35 we detail the results from the same analysis of the mortality statistics from the voters' roll.

Table 35. Ratio of deaths for different age cohorts to deaths among those aged 50+, by year and sex

	Ratio							
Year	female				male			
	20-29	30-39	40-49	20-49	20-29	30-39	40-49	20-49
1999	0.21	0.27	0.21	0.69	0.20	0.32	0.31	0.83
2000	0.23	0.31	0.22	0.76	0.20	0.35	0.33	0.87
2001	0.24	0.34	0.23	0.81	0.19	0.36	0.34	0.89
2002	0.25	0.39	0.26	0.90	0.19	0.40	0.35	0.94
2003	0.24	0.43	0.28	0.94	0.18	0.42	0.38	0.97

Source: The IEC, 2004e. Calculations by authors.

The ratios generated from the voters' roll are generally slightly lower when compared with the figures presented by Dorrington above. This might be explained by the groups of people that our IEC data excludes (as mentioned above). The similarities are more striking however. The IEC data show that the mortality ratio for the younger population increasingly approximates that of the older population, a development that is most pronounced among women, with an increase from 0.69 to 0.94 in the five years. As a reflection of the trend shown in figures 9.4 to 9.6 above, we can see that this increase occurs mainly in the 30-39 age cohort and particularly among women.

So far into the analysis we have clarified what appears to be some worrying trends on the basis of absolute numbers of death among the South African electorate. But we get a better understanding of the different trends that we described above if we also consider whether one of two possible changes in the numbers of registered voters have occurred simultaneously with the changes in the absolute number of mortality:

- The number of registered voters has increased. If such an increase matches the increase in mortality we are simply observing the same relative number of deaths but at a higher level, and there would be no basis for concluding that AIDS-related deaths have affected the electorate at an increasing rate. If an increase corresponds with a decrease in mortality we can conclude that the South African electorate is becoming healthier;
- The number of registered voters has decreased. If such a decrease matches a decrease in mortality we are left with no basis for drawing conclusions about the possible effect of AIDS among the electorate. However, a decrease in numbers of registered voters that corresponds with an increase in mortality among those voters would potentially be particularly problematic as it indicates that the rate of mortality increases among a smaller group of people.

The data from the voters' roll clearly indicate that the number of registered voters has increased in all but the two youngest age cohorts. We need to remember that the numbers on registration that we work with in this chapter do not contradict the information on registration for the 2004 elections that we detailed in chapter eight, since registration campaigns that reportedly were particularly successful in convincing youth to register to vote carried on into 2004.

In table 36 we detail the national figures for the changes in numbers of registered voters that occurred between the end of 1999 and the end of 2003, by age and sex. Two trends are particularly clear. The first is that the number of registered voters increases with an increase in age. This trend was even clearer when the age cohorts 50-59, 60-69, 70-79 and 80+ were looked at separately with an almost 50% increase for the oldest voters. While this of course is a positive trend it is very problematic that there has been a strong downward trend in registration among the younger voters; the number of registered 18-19-year-old men more than halved in four years.

Table 36. Change in numbers of registered voters from 1999 to 2003, per age cohort and sex (%)

Change	Age cohorts				
	18-19	20-29	30-39	40-49	50+
Women	- 49.0	- 10.5	+ 12.7	+ 22.5	+ 23.5
Men	- 54.7	-11.2	+ 13.3	+ 18.3	+ 26.8

Source: IEC, 2004e. Calculations by authors.

Taken as a whole, the number of registered voters increased by 8% in the four years, or by a total of 1 441 977 (from 18 011 064 to 19 453 041). However, as we saw briefly already in figure 6, there was also a 53% increase in the relative number of deaths during the same period, from 1.18% in 1999 to 1.81% in 2003 of the total number of registered voters. It is thus not the case that the increase in absolute numbers of deaths can be explained as "normal" levels of mortality among a higher number of people; the clear trend is that South Africa's voters died at a higher rate in the year preceding the 2004 elections than they did at the time of the 1999 elections. However, as with the trends noted above, this increase also varies significantly between age groups and between men and women. In the figure below, we can see that women between 20 and 49 years of age are particularly affected, with an extraordinary increase of 129% in the relative number of deaths for women 30-39 years old.

Figure 12. Increase (in %) in relative numbers of deaths among registered voters between 1999-2003, per age and sex

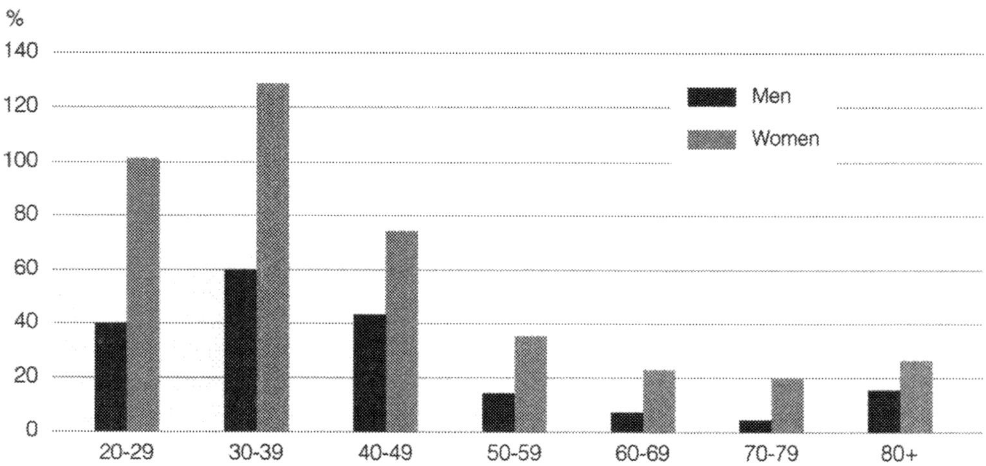

Source: IEC 2004e. Calculations by authors.

To round off this section we can conclude that the mortality profiles that emerge from our analysis of the IEC data from the voters' roll in broad terms match the analyses that Dorrington et al (2001) and Bradshaw et al (2004) present on the basis of the ASSA model and data from the population register respectively, the main findings being that:

- The level of mortality among the South African electorate has increased more between 1999 and 2003 than can be explained by a higher number of registered voters;
- The "mortality profile" is heavily skewed against younger women, with particularly high levels of mortality among women who are 30-39 years old;
- In 2000 and 2003 the demographic aberration occurred that more women than men died in the 20-29 and 30-39 age cohorts respectively, and;
- A second equally problematic trend was that in 2003 mortality among women and men in the age cohort 20-49 had increased to a level where it almost equalled that among those aged 50 years and older (ratios of .94 and .97 respectively).

Given these trends and our analytical framework it would seem that AIDS is the only possible explanation for the increase in mortality according to the "profiles" we have been able to identify, but we shall put that hypothesis to some further tests in section 9.3 below before we formulate any more definite conclusions. First we shall explore a geographic breakdown of the information.

9.2.2 PROVINCIAL AND MUNICIPAL VARIATIONS

We saw in chapter two that the three methods for establishing a national estimate of HIV prevalence, as well as the projections of AIDS mortality based on the ASSA model, all identify a great, albeit somewhat different, variation in the impact of the epidemic in South Africa's nine provinces. If the increase in mortality on the voters' roll that we described above to some degree is caused by AIDS we should expect to see some correlation between these estimates and the provincial "profiles" of mortality in the South African electorate. We shall return to such tests below. Let us first establish what these profiles are by detailing the relative numbers of death across South Africa's provinces and municipalities and how these have changed between 1999 and 2003.

While most of South Africa's municipalities obviously are placed in one of the nine provinces, some municipalities cross provincial boundaries. This complexity is however not reflected in the IEC data set which identifies all municipalities under one province only. This means that where municipalities cross provincial boundaries the change in relative number of deaths will be attributed only to one province. However, while this is important to note for further and more detailed analysis of the data, it should not significantly alter the general trends in the data that we present. In presenting this information we have chosen to focus our attention on the age cohorts of women where we would have expected and also have noticed particularly high levels and increases in mortality: 20-29, 30-39 and 40-

49-year-olds. The corresponding information for other ages and also for men is in some instances available in the appendices.

Figure 13. Relative number of deaths among women in 1999 (in %) by age cohorts and by province

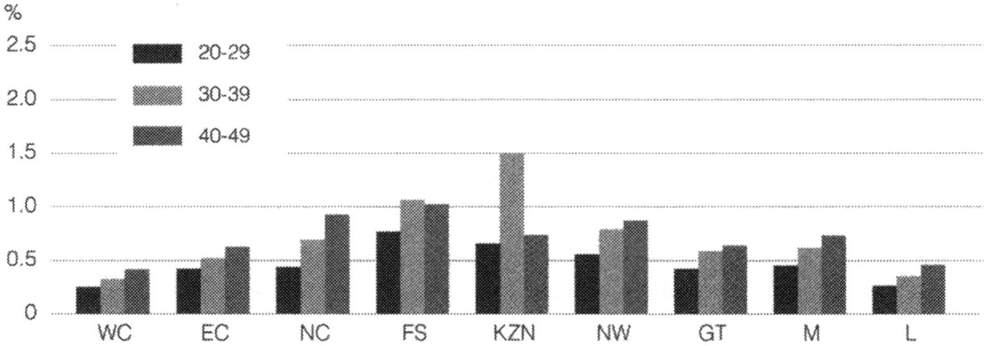

Source: IEC 2004e. Calculations by authors.

Figure 14. Relative number of deaths among women in 2003 (in %) by age cohorts and by province

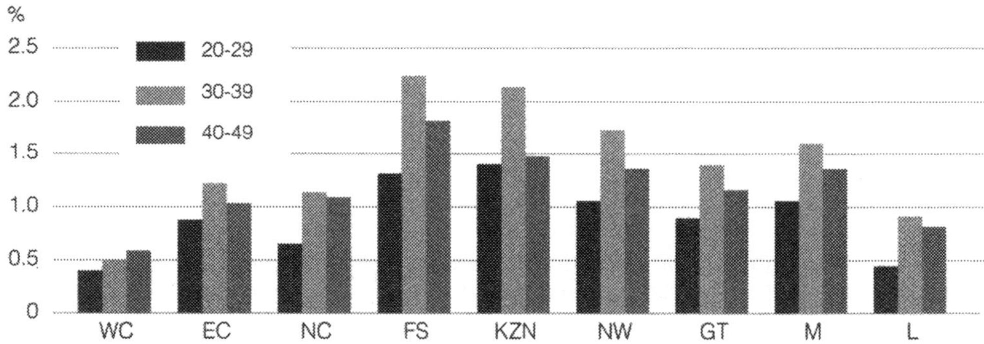

Source: IEC 2004e. Calculations by authors.

The relative number of deaths per province in 1999 placed KwaZulu-Natal clearly at the top of the list, a position it also held on the basis of absolute numbers of deaths (3 502 deaths among 30-39-year-old women). Another observation on the basis of figure 13 is that, with the exception of KwaZulu-Natal and the Free State, mortality was higher among older women than among younger women, as should be expected. By 2003 this pattern had changed quite dramatically, as is shown in figure 14. Not only had the relative numbers of deaths increased in four years, but the "profile" had changed in two important respects. In 2003 it is the Free State that has the highest relative number of deaths among women 30-39 and 40-49 years old, although KwaZulu-Natal, with 11 065 deaths among 30-39-year-old women still dominated the picture in terms of absolute numbers (see further appendix C). A more fundamental change is that by 2003 mortality among 30-39-year-old women had surpassed that of 40-49-year-old women, with the Western Cape being the sole exception.

While we can learn much from the two mortality profiles for 1999 and 2003 that figures 13 and 14 present respectively, it is important to look not only at such "snapshots" in time but also to understand the dynamic of the change in mortality profiles that seems to be underway. One such dynamic aspect concerns the rate at which mortality increased between 1999 and 2003 in the different provinces.

Figure 15. Increase (in %) in the relative numbers of deaths for women, between 1999 and 2003, by age cohort and by province

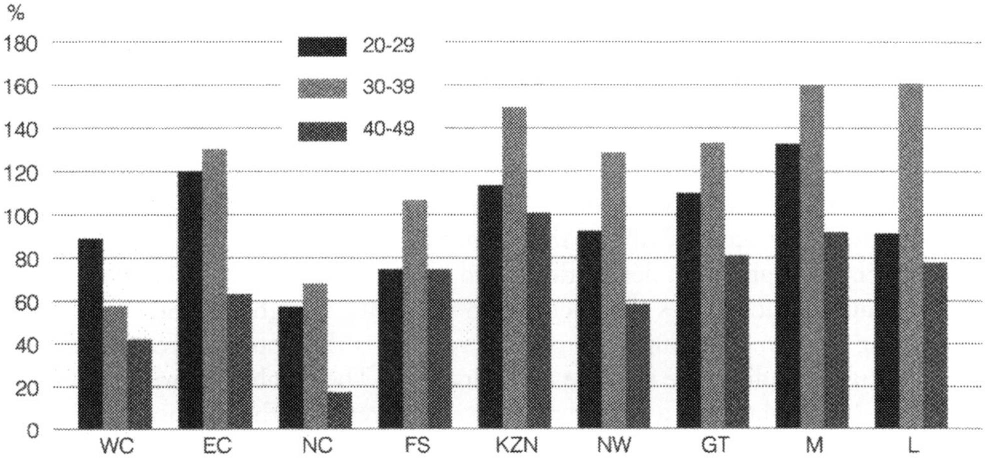

Source: IEC 2004e. Calculations by authors

We can see from figure 15 that it is not in the provinces with the highest mortality in absolute or relative numbers that mortality is experiencing the sharpest increases among registered voters, but in Limpopo and Mpumalanga. Or in other words, whereas KwaZulu-Natal in 2003 had the highest mortality in absolute numbers among women voters aged 30-39 years with 11 065 deaths, and the Free State recorded the highest number of deaths in relative numbers for the same year for women of 30-49 years, the rate at which mortality in relative numbers increased between 1999 and 2003 was highest in Limpopo and Mpumalanga. With increases in the relative numbers of 160.5% and 159.9% respectively for 30-39-year-old women the two provinces are facing a serious challenge to find ways of stopping this trend of sharply rising levels of mortality among some groups of women.

We now turn to describing the mortality profile at a municipal level and we will, as before, focus on registered voters between the ages of 20 and 49. To present the different municipal level profiles effectively we have generated maps of South Africa's municipalities coloured in accordance with a legend that identifies how the relative number of deaths differs between municipalities. The four relevant maps (included at the end of this report) show the increase in the relative number of deaths from 1999 to 2003. The maps are rich in the mass of information they provide, a richness we will not be able to explore fully in this report.[30]

A few features in the municipal profiles are particularly striking, even though the general pattern obviously corresponds with what we know from our analyses.

- The rates of increase in mortality are in some instances alarmingly high. While we noted above that Limpopo was the province with the highest rate of increase in relative number of deaths between 1999 and 2003 at 160% (for women, 30-39 years), such provincial figures contain considerable municipal variations with increases that are more than twice that high. Take for example Lephalale municipality (Ellisras) in the Limpopo province. In 1999 a total of 11 women (30-39 years) died among 4 721 registered voters, a figure that had risen to 57 dead from 5 240 voters in 2003 – an increase in the relative number of deaths of 367%.

- The rates of increase in mortality are in some instances surprisingly low. Even in provinces and areas where adjoining municipalities show high levels of increase in mortality there are single municipalities that appear to have been spared this problematic trend. A good example is the Letsemeng Local Municipality (Koffiefontein) in the Free State. While the province in itself has the highest relative number of deaths among women (30-39 years), an increase that exceeds 250% in the neighbouring Tokologo Local Municipality, the relative number of deaths decreased in the Letsemeng municipality.
- In some municipalities the increase in mortality is higher among men than among women. Although the general pattern is the opposite trend, men are particularly vulnerable in some municipalities. The Thaba Chewu municipality in Mpumalanga is a good example. An increase in the relative number of deaths among women (30-39 years) of 135% between 1999 and 2003 was surpassed by an increase of 241% among registered men of the same age.
- In most municipalities the increase in mortality among women is considerably higher than among men. While we knew this from the analyses above, the differences between the sexes are nevertheless sometimes striking. In Utrecht municipality in KwaZulu-Natal, for example, the relative number of deaths for men (30-39 years) increased by 28% between 1999 and 2003 (seven more deaths among an additional 16 registered voters), while the increase for women of the same age was 343% (21 more deaths among an additional 22 registered voters).

The four features we highlight above of the municipal level mortality profiles of the South African electorate exemplify the mass and complexity of the information that the maps and the original data set contain. It is safe to say that there is no one factor that will explain why we see such variations between the municipalities or between the provinces. Let us therefore explore some of the most likely "suspects" to see how much closer we can get to understanding what causes these patterns in mortality on the South African voters' roll. (See maps in the appendices.)

9.3 A FIRST TAKE ON EXPLAINING THE VARIATIONS

To fully explain a social and demographic "pattern" as complex as the mortality profiles we have described goes far beyond the limits of this report, to the extent it can be done at all. What we will attempt in this section is merely to take the analysis as far as we can at this stage, given the limitations in the data and other resources that have been available to us. Through some initial statistical analysis we hope to establish whether there are any grounds for arguing that two possible and probable causes to the patterns we can observe actually contribute to their explanation: HIV/AIDS and poverty. If either or both of the factors have anything to do with the explanation, we should expect to find correlations between the rate of increase in the relative number of deaths, on the one hand, and levels of poverty and/or the various estimates and projections of HIV and AIDS on the other. Our analysis here will stop at exploring statistical correlations between the variables.[31]

9.3.1 HIV/AIDS

It has been our contention throughout this chapter that the patterns and trends we have described in the mortality rates among the South African electorate are best explained by the HIV and AIDS epidemic. To be more precise, we argue that the particular demographic aberrations we described above – the sharp increases in mortality among registered voters between the ages of 20-49, and particularly among 30-39-year-old women – can to a large extent, if not wholly, be explained by AIDS. We base that argument on the strong correspondence between the "profiles" that our analysis generated and those that have been described by the expert demographers in the field of HIV/AIDS analysis. In this section we shall see if this argument can be further strengthened empirically by establishing correlations between our mortality profiles and the most current estimates of HIV prevalence and projections of AIDS-related illnesses and deaths.

However, since all HIV estimates and AIDS projections are done only on a provincial level, we have to aggregate the mortality data to the same level, hence the cautions noted in section 1.4 also apply here. This aggregation is unfortunate also since it means that we lose information about all the variation between different municipalities in the same province that the maps described so effectively.

Before we discuss the results of the tests we should clarify some of our assumptions that motivate this analysis. The logic of our thinking is as follows. While we do not know the cause of death for any of the deceased individuals who were taken off the voters' roll between 1999 and 2003, our argument that the problematic mortality profiles among 20-49-year-old voters are caused by AIDS-related deaths would be strengthened:

- If the provincial variations in estimates of HIV prevalence by different agencies correlate positively with the provincial variations in increases in the relative number of deaths – *the higher the estimated prevalence of HIV, the higher the number of actual deaths by AIDS*;

- If provincial variations in projections of number of people sick with AIDS correlate positively with the provincial variations in increases in the relative number of deaths – *the higher the projected number of people sick with AIDS, the higher the number of actual deaths by AIDS*;
- If provincial variations in projections of numbers of AIDS-related deaths correlate positively with the provincial variations in increases in the relative number of deaths – *the higher the number of deaths projected to be caused by AIDS, the higher the number of actual deaths by AIDS*.

The results of our tests for correlation are detailed in table 9.3 below. Four salient features of the results are worth further comment. (1) All correlations are positive. The general relationship holds that higher levels of estimated and projected impact of the epidemic correlate with larger increases in mortality, and some of these correlations are exceptionally strong. (2) Some correlations are highly significant. Despite the fact that we are working with few cases, a number of the correlations are nevertheless highly significant. It is obvious that in these cases the "fit" between the estimates and/or projections on the one hand and the increases in mortality on the other is very good indeed (which becomes very clear when the correlation is plotted on the regression line). (3) Some correlations are weaker and not significant. As should be expected, since the various estimates and projections are done for the adults up to the age of 49, the correlations are weaker and not significant for adults older than that. The estimates and projections also do not provide as strong a basis for explanation for women 20-29 years old, perhaps because the actual increase in mortality exceeds expectations. Finally, of the three agencies, the HIV estimates provided by the HSRC through its household survey generate weaker correlations with the actual increases in mortality.

Table 37. Correlating increases in relative number of deaths with HIV/AIDS estimates and projections (N=9)

HIV/AIDS estimates and projections		Age cohort by gender							
		20-29		30-39		40-49		50+	
		female	male	female	male	female	male	female	male
ASSA model	HIV estimate	.514	.948**	.817**	.887**	.830**	.834**	.459	.418
	Sick from AIDS	.285	.890**	.538	.790*	.725*	.691*	.228	.426
	Dead from AIDS	.548	.919**	.719*	.845**	.840**	.836**	.492	.569
Department of Health		.581	.908**	.644	.771*	.751*	.808**	.435	.616
HSRC		.411	.719*	.359	.709*	.641	.687*	.058	.580

Sources: IEC, 2004e; Dorrington, 2001; DoH, 2002; Shisana, 2002.

The table details the correlation coefficients (Pearson's r) between the increases in relative number of deaths between 1999 and 2003 per gender and per age cohort and three different estimates of HIV infection (ASSA model, DOH and HSRC), one projection of AIDS-related sickness (stage 4 of the decease) and one projection of AIDS-related deaths (ASSA model). All data and estimates are on the level of provinces. * Indicates significance at 0.05 level, ** indicates significance at 0.01 level.

On the whole, we would argue, these initial statistical tests provide further validation of our argument that the profiles of mortality we have described above are indeed caused by the HIV/AIDS epidemic among the South African electorate. These tests do not allow us to say anything of the strength of that relation, or about how it should be understood to interact with other factors that have an impact on levels of mortality. We leave this to be explored in future research publications. In the next section we present a similar explorative analysis of our second plausible and potentially complementary explanation – poverty.

9.3.2 POVERTY

In academic and in political debates on the nature, cause and impact of the epidemic the issue of poverty always features, at the very least, as a factor that aggravates the effects of the epidemic and provides conditions that are conducive to the further spread of the virus. On the assumption that our data on mortality actually reflects the impact of AIDS on the South African electorate, in line with our argument in the section above, we can test to what extent this general understanding about poverty in the context of the epidemic has an empirical foundation in our data, again at the level of the nine provinces. As we did above we shall test for correlations between the levels of increase in the relative numbers of deaths and three poverty indicators – income poverty, the Human Development Index (HDI) and the Human Poverty Index (HPI) – as they are defined and measured by the United Nations Development Programme (UNDP) (see chapter two). Given that we work with only nine cases, the same caveats around the statistical analysis apply here as was noted for the preceding section. Mirroring the analyses from section 9.3.1, we would thus say that the data confirms the understanding that poverty is closely linked to the impact of the epidemic:

- If provincial variations in the HPI correlate positively with provincial variations in the increase of relative numbers of deaths – *people die at a higher rate in provinces that have a higher score on the HPI*;
- If provincial variations in the HDI correlate negatively with provincial variations in the increases of relative numbers of deaths – *people die at a lesser rate in provinces that have a higher score on the HDI*;
- If provincial variations in income poverty correlate positively with provincial variations in the increase of relative numbers of deaths – *people die at a higher rate in provinces with a higher percentage of people earning below the poverty line.*

The results of the statistical analysis are somewhat less striking than those for HIV/AIDS. The main result is that, of the three poverty indicators, it is the more complex HPI that provides the best basis for an explanation of the variations in mortality. Our analysis suggests that the combination of the four poverty indicators that make up the HPI – ie the probability at birth of not surviving to age 40; the adult literacy rate; the percentages of people not using improved water sources; and children under five who are underweight – provide a basis for arguing that poverty can account for some of the explanation of the variation in the increase in mortality for the three age cohorts within the age span 20-49. The exception, yet again, is the youngest group of women. The two other poverty indicators are less successful as explanations. While the HDI generates negative correlations as was expected, these are all weaker than the HPI and none is significant. The somewhat simplistic indicator "income poverty" was even more unsuccessful.

Table 38. Correlating increases in relative numbers of deaths with poverty indicators (N=9)

	Age cohorts by gender							
Poverty indicators	20-29		30-39		40-49		50+	
	female	male	female	male	female	male	female	male
Human Poverty Index	.538	.823**	.829**	.755*	.694*	.762*	.530	.256
Human Development Index	-.223	-.401	-.674*	-.430	-.352	-.393	-.423	.214
Income Poverty	-.039	.210	.305	.124	.024	.089	.147	-.404

Source: IEC, 2004e; UNDP, 2003.

Our initial statistical tests provide the basis for arguing, in line with theoretical hypotheses, that both the HIV/AIDS epidemic and poverty has something to do with the explanation of the variations between the provinces in the increases in relative number of deaths.[32]

CONCLUSION

Our analysis in this chapter has, arguably, established a number of important facts and strengthened some arguments. The profiles of mortality among the South African electorate establishes beyond doubt that South Africans are dying according to a pattern that clearly deviates from what should be normal for a population like the South African one. Young men should die at a higher rate than young women and old people should die at a considerably higher rate than young people. But this is not the case in South Africa: in 2003 female voters 20-39 years of age died in higher numbers than their male counterparts and voters below 50 years of age died at almost the same rate as those 50 years of age and older. The rate of the increase in mortality between 1999 and 2003 among 30-39-year-old women is a particular cause for concern. With increases of around 160% in two provinces and municipal increases twice as steep, South Africa is looking at a trend in mortality that should be a cause for the utmost alarm, mobilising a strong response from the whole of society and its political representatives.

Our interpretation was framed by analyses that suggest that these abnormal mortality profiles are caused by AIDS-related deaths to a large extent. Indeed, our comparisons with previous analyses in this literature – analyses that are based both on projections from computer modelling and from "straightforward" analyses of actual deaths on the Population Register – show that mortality on the voters' roll displays the same general features. On this basis alone we conclude that our findings from a new and independent data set of actual deaths corroborate previous analyses and their conclusions. But we took one step further in our analysis and found that the variations in increases in mortality on a provincial level showed substantial correlation with the variations within various estimates and projections of HIV prevalence, as well as sickness and deaths from AIDS. These tests, arguably, further strengthen our argument that the HIV and AIDS epidemic is causing the abnormal mortality profiles to some degree. We could show that poverty – when measured as the HPI – also might provide some explanation. Further statistical analyses and more elaborate theoretical work will explore how the two factors interact more precisely.

When we take a step back from the findings in this chapter we are reminded of the Kenyan nurse and her pessimistic premonition: Forget about elections. All the voters will be dead! While we have established here that South African voters die according to patterns that should not be, we are not raising the same banner as the nurse. Instead we argue (and we imagine she would agree) that it is never too late to address the issue through strong social and political interventions. In line with our general argument in this report we would say that, if anything, the information we have presented here should present voters with an additional incentive to take an active part in democratic elections since they can either put pressure on governments to adjust their policies to really address people's concerns, or exercise their right to select alternative policies by entrusting new mandates to fresh representatives.

The sense of stigma, it seems, is strongest among people who are symptomatic. Respondents argued that most members of the communities would not stand in the same queue with someone with visible signs of the disease, eg body rashes and sores.

CHAPTER 10

TO VOTE OR NOT TO VOTE? EXAMINING THE ROLE OF STIGMA AND DISCRIMINATION IN ELECTIONS

...even though we are suffering from this disease, we know that life is still continuing ... and if we take good care of ourselves, we can live for a long time... – Rural African male,18-24 years, Nongoma.

10.1 INTRODUCTION

We have taken an exploratory and descriptive excursion through a range of issues relating to HIV/AIDS and its effects on governance processes and we have unfurled new insights and considered the central concepts in the previous nine chapters with due attention to both structural and attitudinal factors affecting electoral processes in the context of HIV/AIDS.

Public opinion data from the Afrobarometer survey have provided us with a snapshot in time of generalised public perceptions on the effects of the pandemic and the political dynamic introduced by it. This chapter, in many ways, adds a human face to the analysis. Put another way, it is the embodiment of our critical awareness of the limitations and impersonal nature of statistics in general. The use of multiple sources of data has obviously allowed for the triangulation of this research. Focus group discussions in this regard, as the fourth and last segment of our methodology, lend themselves to deeper qualitative analysis. Our appraisal of people who have had practical experience of the problem we are studying constitutes a fundamental component of the research, as we finally begin to attempt to understand the inter-relationship between those affected by the pandemic and their capacity to participate in elections.

The examination of HIV/AIDS and electoral data has been instructive in determining the unit of analysis. Evidently, the people most affected by the pandemic for reasons cited in chapter two are black registered voters who are living with HIV/AIDS or are care givers. Black people are not only the hardest hit by HIV/AIDS, they also constitute the largest segment of the voting population in South Africa. As a consequence of the legacy of apartheid they also form the most economically disadvantaged group in the country.

As the interaction between poverty and HIV/AIDS has been duly dealt with in the preceding chapters, our intention in this chapter is to focus on the personal experiences of registered voters affected by and infected with HIV/AIDS in South African society. This intervention does not pretend to provide a representative sample. Rather it presents readers with a valuable insight into some of the realities of HIV/AIDS as endured by HIV-positive voters and those associated with caring for infected and affected people.

We are mindful also of the danger of unwittingly contributing to the stigma and discrimination of certain parts of the South African citizenry by alluding to "high-risk populations". We argue, however, that generalising the research would by itself dilute the gravity of the problem and drown the need for marginalised groups to access much-required support.

We believe further that there is substance in extending the analysis on the impact of HIV/AIDS on political participation to relate not only to the infected but to the care givers as people potentially associated with the same vector of discrimination. Studies by South Africa's Department of Health not only confirm that there is indeed a social stigma directed at people living with HIV and AIDS (PLWHAs) who have disclosed their status but that AIDS discrimination is aimed also at those who associate with people who are known to carry the disease (Jennings et al 2002).

10.1.1 DESIGNING THE FOCUS GROUPS

A total of 68 respondents were selected from among care givers and PLWHAs. All were registered voters. We allowed a preponderance of HIV-positive individuals in the ratio 6:4, the PLWHAs being our main interest. It has to be said that eliciting participation from PLWHAs proved to be more difficult in rural areas and Citizen Surveys, which conducted the field work for Idasa-GAP, solicited the assistance of health workers and counsellors to arrive at a reasonable ratio of participation. Thirty nine of the respondents were PLWHAs and 29 were care givers. Groups were disaggregated along gender lines and in relation to age cohorts, taking into account possibilities that different age groups might have different values and aspirations and to allow more transparent debate. At least 50 percent of the group participated as voters in the 2004 elections. Our central research question was to determine: *To what extent – if at all – does the HIV/AIDS pandemic contribute to participation or non-participation of citizens in electoral processes?* Participants were asked to discuss the following themes:

- Reason for participation/non-participation in the 2004 elections;
- Knowledge of the special vote;
- Perception of change agents/political actors;
- Perception of the IEC;
- Perception of elections.

In total six focus groups were held, in the urban areas of the city of Durban, Inanda and Kwa Mashu, and in the rural enclaves of Nongoma. We opted to select groups from among urban and rural populations in a high prevalence area. KwaZulu-Natal was ideal for this purpose being one of the areas worst hit by the pandemic. In addition, the Geographical Information Systems (GIS) we used to map the mortality rates among registered voters in this study suggest a higher than average number of deaths among both male and female voters in that region.

Table 39 Project GAP

		Aids sufferers		Caregivers				
	Total number of respondents	Total aids sufferers	Age group of aids sufferers	Total caregivers	Age group of caregivers			
					18-24	25-34	35-49	50+
Group 1 Urban females – Inanda	12	7	18-24	5			3	2
Group 2 Urban males – Kwa Mashu	12	7	25-34	5		2	2	1
Group 3 Urban males	11	6	35-49	5		1	4	
Urban total	35	30		15	0	3	9	3
Group 4 Rural females – Nongoma	11	6	25-34	5		2	1	2
Group 5 Rural males – Nongoma	12	7	35-49	5	2	3		
Rural total	33	19		14	2	7	2	3
Total	68	39	0	29	2	10	11	6

10.2 THEORETICAL CONTEXT OF STIGMA

Although it occasionally fuels acts of empathy and solidarity, the HI virus from the time of its discovery in the early 1980s has predominantly precipitated fear, denial, stigma and discrimination. Researchers suggest that the allegorical references to shame, guilt, horror and punishment in relation to HIV/AIDS have tended to aggravate one of the most abhorrent forms of social devaluation in recent memory – stigma (Parker and Aggleton, 2002).

Experts on this subject underline that there is a fundamental linkage between pre-existing stigma and discrimination associated with sexuality, gender, race and poverty and HIV/AIDS-related stigma. Fears of contagion and disease pre-date AIDS and epithets associated with the pandemic, it is argued, contribute to legitimising stigmatisation and discrimination (Parker & Aggleton, 2002).

Historical analysis suggests that contagious diseases such as leprosy and tuberculosis, usually caused sufferers to be rejected by society. Sexually transmitted infections (STIs) are still seen to be profoundly shameful, perhaps because the mode of transmission suggests a transgression of moral values within communities. Unfortunately, modernity has hardly moved societies to be more receptive of people afflicted by epidemics. PLWHAs are just as badly treated in communities in the northern hemisphere as they are in the south.

The tragic case of Gugu Dlamini, a resident of the city of Durban, who paid with her life at the hands of a modern-day lynch mob for disclosing her status on World Aids Day in 1998 (Fredriksson & Kanabus. 2004) epitomises the grotesque form that ignorance-driven social responses to HIV/AIDS might assume when confronted with the realities of the pandemic.

10.2.1 Defining stigma and the link to discrimination and prejudice

But why do HIV and AIDS generate so much stigma and discrimination the world over? What do we understand by stigma? What is the relationship between stigma, discrimination and prejudice? What, in the end, are the probable political, social and cultural consequences of HIV/AIDS-related stigma and discrimination?

Gilmore and Sommerville (1994, in Unicef/Panos, 2002) define stigma as "an attribute used to set the affected person or groups apart from the normalised social order, and this separation implies devaluation". UNAIDS underlines that stigmatisation refers to "a process of devaluation within a particular culture or setting, where certain attributes are seized upon and defined as discredible or not worthy". (Panos/Unicef, 2004). Stigma, it might be inferred, connotes a form of shame arising when established norms, values and sanctions are seen to be contravened by an individual or group. On the other hand, discrimination takes place "when a distinction is made against a person that results in their being treated unfairly and unjustly on the basis of their belonging, or being perceived to belong, to a particular group". In relation to HIV/AIDS it implies that one is unfairly treated on the presumption of, or actual, HIV/AIDS status.[33]

Prejudice is distinguished from discrimination as the latter denotes a form of action. It is argued that prejudice, which is generated by fear, ignorance and deviance, is held within one's mind and only translates into discrimination once one acts on one's negative predisposition (Brown, cited in Jennings et al, 2002). As might be discerned from the definitions, the mark of shame or devaluation (stigma) placed on a person's reputation by prejudiced members of a community tends to determine the extent of exclusion (discrimination) from the rest of the society.

10.2.2 Categorising discrimination

Jennings et al (2002) categorise discrimination in three broad areas: individual, institutional and structural. They posit that at a personal level discrimination is experienced within closely knit personal networks: these include the failure of romantic relations, family ties or friendships due to fear or rejection of a PLWHA. At an institutional level discrimination is said to occur in an institutional setting: PLWHAs are marginalised or excluded from employment, or denied certain positions, insurance, medical aid, access to loans and protection of the law. Finally, at a structural level, societal structures have in-built mechanisms that discriminate against certain groups eg women who are denied inheritance of property or access to information by rural and urban dwellers skewered by structural factors that favour elites in the urban zones. Access to condoms is likewise more likely in urban than rural areas (Jennings et al, 2002).

In the main the body of literature indicates that there are several key levels at, or conditions in, which stigma and discrimination occur in relation to HIV/AIDS:

- Community;
- Legislation;
- Family;
- Employment;
- Health care;
- Gender;
- Race;
- School;
- Class; and
- Media.

Community level. Some of the underlying movers of stigma and discrimination include religious and cultural beliefs, ignorance and racial prejudice. Fredriksson & Kanabus (2004) cite the following perceptions as contributing factors:

- HIV/AIDS is seen as a death sentence;
- Fear of contracting the disease;
- The religious belief that the infected are recipients of God's wrath[34];
- PLWHAs are often thought to be responsible for contracting it; and
- The disease is associated with certain behaviours (prostitution, homosexuality and drug use) (Fredriksson & Kanabus, 2004).

The enduring image of HIV/AIDS as a disease of shame, they argue, is reinforced by authoritative images of AIDS as celestial punishment for immorality; a crime for which there are guilty and innocent actors; a war that must be won; a dreadful illness for which its sufferers are to be feared and isolated. The tendency for people not infected to consider the disease as someone else's problem increases the exclusion of those who are infected and affected. Denial and discrimination are in fact bedfellows, allowing fear and stigma to fester because a condition is perceived to exist only for certain irresponsible people.

In some African societies witchcraft has been cited as the cause of death even where AIDS is clearly known to be the cause. This form of denial arises because witchcraft, as opposed to AIDS, can be managed within the local cosmology and healing systems. Rejection takes on moderate and extreme forms: infected and affected persons will be denied handshakes, bus seats or the sharing of cups and cooking utensils (Panos/Unicef, 2001). Studies also reveal that in India labelling and name-calling of PLWHAs is commonplace (Panos/Unicef, 2001). At the most extreme, they might pay with their lives.

Legislation. Fredriksson and Kanabus (2004) conceive that stigma and discrimination can be accentuated further by legislation which imposes compulsory screening and testing, and restrictions on travel and migration for PLWHAs who are seen as a health risk. The sum effect of statutory sanctions on so-called "high risk groups," they suggest, is to buttress a false sense of security among the uninfected sections of the population. Conversely, perhaps as an outcome of human rights activism, many governments have protected the rights of PLWHAs with regard to accessing employment, education, treatment and support, and maintaining their privacy and confidentiality if necessary. The enforcement of such laws generally leaves much to be desired, judging by the many violations that are reported worldwide.[35] In South Africa, despite legal protection of PLWHAs and therefore some security, experts argue that it is not possible to legislate against prejudice, implying that the discrimination experienced by people known to be HIVpositive persists, despite the law (Heywood, cited in Jennings et al, 2002).

Employment. In the same vein, despite the fact that most countries, including South Africa, forbid pre-employment testing for HIV/AIDS, industry finds ways of establishing the status of its employees, leading to denial of employment or termination. Disclosure at workplaces often consigns the infected person to marginalisation or discrimination and the loss of training and promotional opportunities.[36]

Family. It is documented that even within families PLWHAs are not fully embraced and that non-heterosexual women come off worse than their male counterparts. Verbal abuse, rejection, eviction and imposed restrictions are some of the forms of discrimination manifest in families. There is overwhelming evidence that families constitute the core of care-giving systems, but it also is clear that family systems are over-burdened, lacking in resources, and sick members might be deemed dispensable in the end.

Health care. Discriminatory practices in the health care systems are also likely to exacerbate the problem. Testing without consent, denial of attention for fear of infection,[37] lack of confidentiality[38] and withholding treatment are all fuelled by ignorance or prejudice.

Race and ethnicity. It has been emphasised in more recent studies that race and ethnicity interact with HIV and AIDS-related stigma. The pandemic has been characterised by racist assumptions that "African sexuality" and behaviour are "immoral". The racial veneer over the AIDS pandemic exudes extremely powerful forms of stigma and discrimination (Parker and Aggleton, 2002).

Gender. The unfortunate position of women in many countries is one of the most critical factors in stereotyping and therefore discrimination. Economically, culturally and socially disempowered, women are depicted as prostitutes who are responsible for the spread of the disease. A Panos/Unicef report[39] reveals that women are often less likely to disclose their status for fear of divorce, violence or further disclosure. The fate of Gugu Dlamini might be understood in this context.

Schools. School systems are guilty also of discharging infected learners; HIV-positive teachers are forced to withdraw from public life for fear of taunts. Studies in Zambia showed that children whose parents were known to have died of AIDS were often bullied. The National Association of Social Workers in the United States also cite a case where local school boards refused to enrol HIV-positive children. They lament that courts are "steadily chipping away" at the protections afforded to HIV-positive individuals under the Americans with Disabilities Act (ADA).[40]

Class. Our discussion on electoral systems underlines the fact that AIDS is not a problem only for the poor judging by the rate of death among middle-aged politicians. Politicians will face the same societal responses, including campaign-related slander, once they disclose their status; this also is likely to drive them into silence and make them less able to communicate effective messages to the populace. However, studies by the Department of Health indicate that people of higher social class are less likely to suffer the same extent of discrimination.

Media. Stereotyping through media messages, terminology and a focus on certain types of behaviours by particular groups of people might add to stigmatisation and discrimination.

10.2.3 DISCRIMINATORY ATTITUDES IN SOUTH AFRICA

The Department of Health reports in its 2002 study that discrimination "is quite high and widespread" in the country (Jennings et al, 2002).

> *It would appear that human rights are not widely appreciated or respected. Furthermore, it appears that it is the level of education of a respondent that most seems to influence their attitudes (Jennings et al, 2002).*

Attempting to illustrate discrimination among the citizenry, the department conducted focus group discussions, maintaining homogeneity in relation to age, race and gender, with participants drawn from metropolitan and rural areas. The survey focused on interviews with black (African) populations (for lack of resources to conduct more comprehensive studies) in the east Rand metropolitan municipality in Gauteng and the Nongoma area in KwaZulu-Natal. Of a total of 501 respondents, 343 were female. Opinions were sought on a range of statements that generally teased out individual positions on such things as:

- The right of PLWHAs to have children;
- Whether PLWHAS should have separate hospital facilities;
- Whether media images should portray PLWHAs leading normal lives;
- Whether there must be compulsory pre-employment testing;
- Whether the names of PLWHAs should be publicised;
- Whether PLWHAs should be restricted or not allowed to work;
- Whether PLWHAs should be separated from others.

What is clearly indicative of the extent of discrimination are the high numbers of people who seemed to support compulsory testing (22% separate hospital facilities for PLWHAs (26%) and prohibition of child-bearing amongst PLWHAs (84%), see table on the following page.

10.2.4 LEVELS OF DISCRIMINATION

The study found that there was a higher degree of discrimination among rural than among urban dwellers and level of education and exposure to information on HIV/AIDS is a considered explanation for this variance.

> *While one in five (20%) urban residents displayed a high level of discrimination, this proportion was far higher at one in three (34%) rural residents. One could surmise that the differences reflect the differential access*

to campaigns and resources dealing with HIV/AIDS (Jennings et al, 2002:27).

Table 40. Level of discrimination by age, employment status and area of dwelling

		Low (%)	Medium (%)	High (%)
All respondents		37	36	27
Age	18-35	42	35	23
	36-55	31	38	31
	56+	33	33	33
Employment status	Employed	51	32	17
	Unemployed	34	38	28
Area of dwelling	Urban	48	31	20
	Rural	25	40	34

Source: Jennings *et al*, 2002

The study is instructive in informing us of just how these statements on discrimination could possibly impact on an individual seeking participation in formal public processes such as elections. The fact that 47% of the respondents said they would not disclose their status to colleagues demonstrates perhaps the apprehension that accompanies the knowledge of one's status. Thirty seven percent of the respondents in this research would not tell friends and only 17% would withhold information of their status to family. There obviously is a preponderance of people who are less inclined to disclosure and, taking into account that the DOH did not seek to know the HIV status of its respondents, this might help us connect with the sentiments of people who care for AIDS orphans and HIV/AIDS sick, but who are not themselves infected. Also of note is the high numbers of respondents who were fearful of contracting the disease (55%) and those who believed HIV/AIDS was due to deviant behaviour (65% and 8%) in medium and high categories respectively). While it was not clear from the findings if the level of fear translated into increased discriminatory attitudes, it was generally concluded that lower levels of fear contributed to decreased discrimination.

With an increasing number of people experiencing personal loss, with more citizens enduring the pandemic as a personal problem, with the burden of orphans compromising the capacity of households to cope and of care givers to lead normal lives, how do these fears of contracting HIV/AIDS play themselves out in the political arena?

10.3 FINDINGS

We reiterate that the reflections of PLWHAS and care givers in this Idasa-GAP study merely provide a view into how people afflicted by HIV/AIDS and their care givers interact with electoral processes. The analysis is subjective and therefore will not necessarily illustrate the extent of the impediments to voting inherent within the local communities; rather it is indicative of the nature and some of the causes of disconnection from or connection to political activity. In the main we seek answers to broad points of inquiry and to specific election-related queries:

- Are the respondents active political actors?
- Has their HIV/AIDS in any way compromised their ability and capacity to engage in political life?
- Are they less able now than before to connect with change agents?
- Is their enthusiasm for politics diminished or stimulated by their potentially life-threatening condition?
- Were they able to participate in the 2004 elections and did they access the special vote?
- To what extent, if at all, does caring for orphans affect their ability to vote?
- Do they get a sense that elections will change their quality of life?

10.3.1 THE PRINCIPLE OF UNIVERSAL ADULT SUFFRAGE

The nature of elections and their importance to the discourse on democratisation has been well underlined in the preceding chapters. We reiterate the fact that the process of elections allows the greatest possible number of adult citizens to select their choice of policy (including HIV/AIDS policy) through the ballot. It is essential that such processes are free and that they are devoid of fear, intimidation, violence or discrimination of all sorts. The full participation of all citizens in electoral processes is an underlying principle embraced by the continent of Africa in its goal of fulfilling universal adult suffrage and sustaining democracy. It is implied in the declarations below that to the greatest extent possible, nation states must endeavour to facilitate the expression of the will of all eligible voters on public affairs.

The principles are endorsed by no less an authority than the African Union in its Election Guidelines, the Southern African Development Community (SADC) in its Mauritius Charter of 2004 and the SADC Parliamentary Forum in its election norms and standards.[41] The notion of universal adult suffrage is inclusive rather than exclusive and therefore prioritises the realisation of full political rights over narrow political considerations.

In this regard there is nothing to even remotely allude to the exclusion of PLWHAs from accessing the special vote in the Electoral Act 33 (1) (a) of South Africa (EISA, 2004). The question therefore is whether the people who deem themselves disadvantaged are willing and able to participate in elections, taking all environmental and structural factors into consideration.

KNOWLEDGE OF THE SPECIAL VOTE

One of the key determinants of participation in elections is the availability of information on civic and voting rights. Voter and civic education, in this sense, play a catalytic role in stimulating citizen interest in the electoral process.

It appears voter education campaigns by the IEC and particularly information on the special vote were effective as the majority of the respondents in all six groups in this study confirmed having heard of it. Media coverage in South Africa is quite extensive with the availability of private, public and community broadcasting services, in addition to multilingual print products.[42] It is hardly surprising that in the Afrobarometer October 2000 comparative study entitled Views of Democracy in South Africa and the Region: Trends and Comparisons, South Africans are said to "have the highest levels of access to political information through various forms of news media" (Mattes, 2000).

IEC INFORMATION OUTREACH

The primary responsibility for voter education and information in South Africa falls squarely on the IEC, in terms of the Electoral Commission Act (EISA, 2004). Based on its assessment of competences and capacity to comply to its standards, the IEC may assign voter education and information outreach functions to accredited voter educators. Political parties and NGOs are permitted also to perform additional voter education functions. Election observer reports indicate that the IEC did work closely with media outlets to relay election information via live debates, special articles, news items and voter education drama series through the electronic and print media. NGOs such EISA and IDASA also produced targeted voter education material in conjunction with the IEC. There seems no doubt that information in the electoral process culminating in the 2004 polls was reasonably sufficient (EISA, 2004).

Indeed a snapshot in the KwaZulu-Natal areas we surveyed is indicative of a fairly elaborate information outreach programme. Respondents in our focus group discussions report that radio and television, newspapers reinforced by posters and loudhailers were the primary and secondary sources of information accessed by respondents in the IDASA-GAP focus groups respectively. But while the IEC was the originator of the messages, the carry-on effect, respondents say, was achieved by other agents, particularly political parties and traditional leaders. Most importantly the rounds done by councillors, indunas and kingships to educate the masses appear to have reached constituencies in the locations of this study. School systems and home visits by IEC officials and party loyalists also were mentioned as sources of information on the special vote.

The respondents confirmed that none had heard any specific reference by the IEC to the eligibility of PLWHAs for the special vote. And none of the respondents apparently used the special voting mechanism. We found a sense of uncertainty among the respondents as to whether people with AIDS could motivate for the use of the special vote. One respondent said he waited for an IEC official to come to help an ill family member, but the official did not turn up; so he and the relative did not vote. Although not clearly expressed, we surmise that the respondents would use the special vote if it were explicitly mentioned that they were eligible. Informed members of the groups, for example, expressed strong opinions to the effect that the IEC does not specifically target HIV-positive people and care givers and should do so to promote their participation in political life. This is due to the high perceptions of stigma and discrimination that respondents feared would accompany their interaction with the greater community in an electoral environment. Minority sentiments reflected the despair and resignation that comes with infection:

> *...when a person finds out they are HIV positive, they can't see anything else in front of their eyes other than death. So even voting becomes pointless because why should I bother if I am dying anyway...?* – Urban African male, 18-24yrs Kwa Mashu.

A few respondents confused the IEC with the government. This confusion manifested itself through continuous reference to the IEC's supposed responsibility for the treatment of PLWHAs! At least one respondent expressed total ignorance of what the IEC was.

DO ELECTIONS HOLD ANY VALUE FOR PLWHAS AND CARE GIVERS?

> *They are still people too and they are still alive and healthy...* – Urban African male, 35-49yrs, Umlazi

There was no variance between the younger respondents (18-24) and the older ones (25-49) in respect of their desire to be involved in political activities including elections: It would appear that HIV/AIDS did not of itself dampen the political enthusiasm of PLWHAs. Rather the environmental factors within a community played a major role, particularly the extent of stigma and discrimination, which we shall deal with later in this section. The extent of illness in the main would pre-determine the degree of enthusiasm to override any perceived prejudice among the community and engage in public voting.

Some of the reasons expressed by the respondents for non-participation in elections echo the sentiments of citizens who are not infected. The younger group (18-24) was more emphatic in relating non-participation to broken political promises, for instance. These expressions would not be any different from those of an uninfected ordinary citizen of the same voting age.[43]

It would seem, however, that PLWHAs were more likely to take part in elections if they had not publicly declared their status or if they do not exhibit any symptoms of AIDS. But that would depend largely on whether they are in an urban or rural setting. We had stronger and more consistent references to stigma and discrimination from the rural-based groups than their urban counterparts. There is a strong corroboration with other studies on stigma and discrimination, such as the DOH research of 2002, which places rural-based South Africans at the receiving end of most AIDS-related discrimination.

With respect to other forms of participation, some respondents claimed to be involved in local rallies and campaign activities or at least expressed an interest in being politically active. Care givers tended to find political activities time consuming, while some of the PLWHAs thought they were potentially damaging should their status be unduly exposed beyond known family circles.

SALIENT POINTS

The most dominant opinion among the PLWHAs and care givers interviewed in this study suggests that elections are viewed with utmost importance by the majority of both infected and affected persons. The fact that the respondents are African or black, perhaps, is of critical importance as this is the section of the population that had been denied rights for more than a century by successive pre-apartheid and apartheid administrations. It stands to reason that they would harbour a more intense need to vote.

Among the larger pool of respondents, voting was closely related to change or high expectations of change in personal and societal circumstances. Respondents gave a number of reasons for voting or wanting to vote: A reference to tangible improvements in life in general was made but aspirations to greater political dividends also were expressed. These included:

- Relatively more job opportunities and access to pension funds generated by a democratically elected government (see chapter nine);
- Improved access to water and sanitation;
- Improved road and housing infrastructure;
- Greater availability of health services, electricity and other social welfare benefits.

However, there were also negative factors that moved some participants to seek participation in elections: This body of opinion suggests that the supposed strides in improvements to social welfare since the advent of democracy in 1994 must be measured against the perceived failures, such as the alleged inability to arrest the spread of corruption in high places. Voting, they said, gave ordinary citizens power to put in place a political party with a policy that would benefit the disadvantaged.

WHY PLWHAs AND CARE GIVERS MIGHT NOT VOTE

That all groups hold some relative regard for elections seems to be a well expressed opinion. However, the flip-side of this explains why people who should have voted opted out. Because there was a more emotive discussion on this topic by participants it is necessary to divide the factors that cause people not to vote into two: 1) attitudinal and 2) structural.

Attitudinal refers to factors that would cause PLWHAs and care givers not to participate in elections due to the negative pre-dispositions (real or imagined) of the community towards them.

Structural factors relate to logistical arrangements put in place to facilitate processing of electors; it includes natural barriers, such as distance and time.

ATTITUDINAL FACTORS

- Stigma and discrimination;
- Political disillusionment;
- Reacting to physical health circumstances (personal or anothers); and
- Contending priorities (care for orphans Vs elections).

> *There was a lady in Kwa Mashu ... they killed her because she told them that she was positive.* – Urban African female, 35-49yrs, Umlazi

Stigma and discrimination resonated as the single most dominant determinant for lack of participation in elections. The PLWHAs harboured seemingly well founded fears that communities would ostracise or marginalise them further if they exposed themselves to major public events. Some described their status as "a serious issue", the knowledge of which is better confined to family and close relatives.

The respondents' opinions correlate with the findings of studies on stigma and discrimination, particularly the DOH's, that HIV/AIDS remains a taboo amongst South African communities, especially in the rural enclaves. The sense of stigma, it seems, is strongest among people who are symptomatic. Respondents argued that most members of the communities would not stand in the same queue with someone with visible signs of the disease eg body rashes and sores. Worse still, some suggested weight loss from any kind of disease was easily construed to be AIDS-related and therefore even people who did not know their status would eschew participation for fear of being mistaken for a PLWHA.

Some care givers tending to sick relatives or to AIDS orphans were similarly apprehensive of participation in public affairs: Mere association with AIDS sick or AIDS orphans might also cause them to become targets of discrimination, they argued.

Political disillusionment: It is significant perhaps to note that it is the younger group, particularly urban males in the 18-24 age cohort, who alluded to the fact that PLWHAs should be given special job considerations to motivate them to participate in politics. It is significant also to note that of the six groups, all the 12 respondents in the 18-24 groups of urban males had voted. This might be explained if we assume that mortality from AIDS has generally occurred in the age cohorts 30-39 years, then the 18-24 group is possibly the healthier and more energetic group, hence their very expectant approach to life. There is obviously an indication here that the younger urban respondents are more critical but also have greater aspirations for change. Being urbanites, they also might have greater access to information on campaign issues, including the availability of treatment programmes and government responsibilities in that regard.[44] It is this group that seemed to demand more services for PLWHAs from government including education; larger budget allocations for treatment, care and support; and special employment considerations. Generally, all groups converged on the notion that HIV/AIDS is primarily "a government problem" but that communities and families also had some responsibilities in alleviating the conditions of PLWHAs and orphans.

> *I think they (politicians) talk about HIV and they lie about it. They are just trying to get people's votes and they have been talking about it for years now but they have done nothing about it.* – Rural African female, 35-49yrs Nongoma.,

ILL HEALTH, ORPHANS

> *(Why didn't you vote?) I was sick and I couldn't walk.* – Rural African male 18-24yrs Nongoma..

Personal illness and care giving came through as important determinants of whether one participates in elections or not. Male participants in the 18-24 cohort and females in the 25-49 age bands emphasised their personal state of physical health, and attendance to sick relatives or orphans, as major impediments to participation. Persons who had AIDS-related complexes were least likely to expose themselves at public events such as elections, it was learnt. Several respondents considered voting stations as "places of gossip".

Chores associated with care giving, such as drawing water, finding food for the ill and orphaned children, and gardening, occupy more importance in the hierarchy of their priorities, according to the care-givers in the 35-49 age band, who called for the voting period to be longer than two days to allow them to participate.

> *I had registered to vote but on the day I had a problem with the AIDS orphans that I look after. The thing is I live with my three boys and the one is very young and I couldn't leave him with the others who are also young.* – Urban African male, 18-24yrs, Kwa Mashu.

Some respondents reported that because most political rallies took place on Sundays, their favoured day of prayer, they would elect religious events rather than political activities. This might be explained by the trust PLWHAs have expressed in church ministers and clerics, who often provide much-needed counselling services and allow them to escape momentarily from a life of despair and rejection.

STRUCTURAL FACTORS

In addition to societal attitudes respondents mentioned logistical or structural factors as contributing to non-participation:

- Lack of toilet facilities;
- Lack of water;
- Lack of seating facilities;
- Long queues; and
- Lack of transport.

Lack of toilet facilities and water. A recurring viewpoint among the groups was that failure to participate in elections by PLWHAs was accentuated by the limited (or lack of) toilet and water facilities at polling stations. The overbearing opinions in this regard indicated that people who had AIDS tended to be afflicted by diarrhoeal diseases and would require regular visits to the toilet/bathroom. In the absence of running water such regularity would generate embarrassment, gossip and discrimination. Although this study did not have the capacity to investigate the availability or state of ablution facilities at all polling stations, it would appear that it was more a concern for the rural folk, particularly the 24-49 female participants.

Transport and seating facilities. To a lesser extent, transport and lack of chairs were cited also as problems for PLWHAs. Although the average distance between homesteads and voting stations was 7.5-8km in urban and 12.5-13km in rural areas, according to the IEC, some participants felt people afflicted by debilitating illnesses should get the benefit of free transport to the polls. Other participants felt also that the lack of chairs discouraged them from voting because they could not possibly stand for long owing to ill health. Alternatively, it was suggested by a few that the sick should be allowed to vote from home. The younger voters (18-24) provided perhaps one of the discordant perspectives to the discourse by alluding to the fact that distance was not a problem and that queues were processed relatively expeditiously in the 2004 general elections. A number of them cited misplaced identity cards, ignorance of the special vote and power relations between the sexes in households that pre-determined involvement in the polls.

> *I was sick on the voting line and they said that I could not sit on the benches they had for the elderly and sick people. I told them I was not feeling well and they said I was not telling the truth.* – HIV-positive rural African female, 35-49yrs, Nongoma

STIGMA AND DISCRIMINATION AS BARRIERS TO POLITICAL PARTICIPATION

But perhaps the most striking factor to come out of these discussions is the reference to stigma and discrimination as probably the most compelling issue for non-participation. The salient factor here is that depending on the levels of discrimination in their communities, PLWHAs are less inclined to vote if they have publicly disclosed their HIV status. The rural respondents especially expressed profound fears of isolation and rejection. The generalised comments from respondents point to the possibilities that people with visible marks of illness or who had openly disclosed their status were prime targets of such discrimination or even violence.

Apparently, even people with an illness such as malaria, in which weight is lost, can be assumed to have HIV/AIDS by ignorant members of especially rural communities, who might equate weight loss to the effects of the pandemic. The concerns about stigma were, again, more glaring among rural participants than their urban counterparts.

The respondents who voted in the 2004 elections were not oblivious to the perceived dangers of being HIV positive. (It cannot be ascertained from the discussions whether all of the respondents who voted had not disclosed their status publicly.) We do get an overall impression though that, in the main, the majority of the voters in the focus groups were comfortable to participate in voting partly due to the non-(public)-disclosure of their status.

Who are the likely change agents?

While the situation of PLWHAs and care givers, from their own accounts, does not amount to desperation, it does in a way expose the gulf between them and their elected representatives. Apart from attributing the acquisition of knowledge of the special vote to party agents in some cases, there is no mention of political leaders as "saviours" or the main change agents in regard to the situation of PLWHAs and care givers. When the respondents were asked directly who they thought was most likely to give them a voice in the political arena and respond favourably to their dire circumstances, religious leaders and television stars came top of the list in all groups except the 18-24 urban males (who prioritised politicians, which can perhaps be expected as they were also the keenest voters). Community leaders and counsellors were next in line.

Overall politicians were viewed as potentially pivotal in dealing with stigma and discrimination, but usually unfulfilling of their electioneering promises. We can understand the choice of local religious leaders in both rural and urban enclaves because much comfort for ostracised people has been sought from the churches. Although some clerics are guilty of projecting HIV/AIDS as a form of punishment from God, it might be inferred from the discussions that the sick and rejected do seek and find solace in prayer extended by local religious groups. Similarly, in close-knit societies of rural South Africa, where people tend to know one another, community leaders might play a key role in educating citizens about their rights and assist in reducing the levels of stigma and discrimination against PLWHAs.

It is underlined by respondents also that the outreach of television and radio and the positive stories about PLWHAs in the national media depicted by celebrities helps them to connect with the positive energy of compassion and solidarity issuing from sections of the nation. Further, the government as an institution is seen to be a strong change agent in terms of its capacity to reach all citizens and educate them on the consequences of stigma and discrimination through its medical professionals. Traditional healers occupy the lowest rating presumably for their deficiencies in terms of outreach.

VISIBILITY OF PLWHAs IN THE POLITICAL ARENA: A MOTIVATING FACTOR

> *When prominent people go and vote and you are sitting at home watching, having already decided not to vote...you can say, hey, there is so and so ... they are HIV-positive just like me ... there he is voting...* – Urban African male, Kwa Mashu.

The varied but often converging opinions of our respondents do not help us to articulate on broader issues around how the PLWHAs would respond as a collective if their demands were not met by the government. However, they do give us discernible consensus through the strongly expressed desire by the majority of how important it is for them to have a voice in the political arena.

Elections provide but one form of participation. Involvement in political campaigning, in community forums and rallies and in government by PLWHAs resonates as perhaps some of the more regular forms of participation that should complement electoral engagement.

The public declaration of an HIV status by political leaders is seen as a fundamental factor in eroding the spectre of HIV/AIDS as a disease of a condemned few, who are often poor and black. A few suggest that South Africa would go a long way to moderating stigma and discrimination if they allowed HIV-positive people to be elected or appointed to high office. This appears to be a way of bridging the perceived gulf between elected officials and PLWHAs, of ensuring that political dividends trickle down to all sections of society, including those infected with and affected by the pandemic. However, they are those who see discrimination playing a role at the highest level:

> *In reality it would not help to say people who are HIV positive who want to campaign for elections should disclose their status because no one would come because people fear AIDS.* – Urban African female, Inanda.

We conclude this section by underlying the sentiment most likely to reflect the discernible consensus of the focus groups: that, like everybody else, PLWHAs value the dividends of democracy and that, given the right conditions, they would, to a great extent, express their will in the electoral arena.

CONTEXTUALISING THE DEMOCRATIC DIVIDENDS : HUMAN DEVELOPMENT INDICATORS

The above discussion would be incomplete without reference to Human Development Indicators which perhaps help us explain the perception of progress, or lack of it, since South Africa became a democracy. We heard some of the voting members of the focus group discussions highlight employment and improved health care, water and sanitation as motivators for participation, despite their status. Others have not been entirely satisfied with the pace of change and they choose to vote in the hope that life will take a dramatic turnaround.

Generally the optimism expressed by the PLWHAs in the importance of elections to their lives can be correlated with the United Nations Development Programme's 2003 Human Development Report (HDR) so we are not simply bound by perceptions but can actually relate to developments on the ground.

IMPROVEMENTS IN EDUCATION SINCE 1994

According to the HDR for South Africa, the delivery of basic services has clearly improved in several areas since 1994. Schools without telephones decreased from 59% (1996) to 36.4% (2000); the percentage of schools without running water decreased from 34% to 27%; the percentage of students without access to proper toilet facilities declined from 55% (6.6 million students in 1996) to 16% (1.9 million students in 2000); access to electricity improved from 40% to 54.9% in all schools; and the number of schools with computers increased from 2 241 to 6 581. The transformation of the education system since 1994 has brought several achievements, including:

- The creation of a single national Department of Education out of 19 racially, ethnically and regionally divided "departments of education";
- The creation of non-discriminatory school environments with access based on criteria other than race or religion. Delivery of certain basic services has clearly improved and remains at high levels.

KwaZulu-Natal, like all other provinces, has benefited from these developments as indicated in table 41.

Table 41. Performance of the provincial departments in the delivery of stationery (2001-2002)

	2001	2002
	% of stationery delivered*	% of stationery delivered*
Eastern Cape	53%	varied 45%-88%**
Free State	98%	100%
Gauteng	98%	varied 45%-88%**
KwaZulu-Natal	31%	97% (all schools covered)
Mpumalanga	100%	100% (all schools covered)
Northern Cape	90%	100% (all schools covered)
Limpopo	95%	90% (96% of schools covered)
North West	98%	100%
Western Cape	89%	85.90%

Source:UNDP, 2003: 23.

* % delivered per order. ** Varies according to school district.

IMPROVEMENTS IN HEALTH CARE

South Africa's HDR (pp 28-31) also illustrates headway in the health sector since the democratically elected government assumed power in 1994. From 14 health authorities under apartheid South Africa, the new government began to consolidate the health system under one umbrella body, the national Department of

Health. At the heart of the restructuring of the apartheid health system was the introduction of primary health care through the district health system. A strong focus on rural health programmes under the Reconstruction and Development Programme (RDP) brought services or made commitments to bring health facilities to rural areas, informal settlements and unserviced areas. The government also has indicated that by 2004 all clinics will have basic minimum standards of service. In addition there are more than 4 000 clinics, 2 298 of which have been upgraded since 2001 through programmes like the Clinic Upgrading and Building Programme (CUBP). Primary capital allocations to health, provided under the Hospital Facilities Revitalisation Grant, also made additional funds available for the construction of three major hospitals, Durban Academic Hospital, Umtata Hospital and Pretoria Academic Hospital.

HOUSING DELIVERY

Quoting the Department of Housing (2003), the HDR reports that about 1.5 million houses were completed between 1994 and 2003. Between 28% and 54% of all housing subsidies approved were given to women-headed households, depending on the province.

It is interesting to note that at 256 542 units KwaZulu-Natal is the second-highest beneficiary after Gauteng (356 556) in terms of the total number of housing units developed between 1994 and 2003. It might explain the perceptions of improvements indicated by a majority of the respondents.

Table 42. Number of houses completed (1994-2003)

	1994-96	1997	1998	1999	2000	2001	2002	2003	Total
Eastern Cape	6 511	32 223	24 659	20 345	34 021	10 816	58 662	7 449	194 686
Free State	13 042	18 001	17 391	7 177	16 088	7 005	9 155	3 371	91 230
Gauteng	56 239	70 924	58 170	45 384	38 547	46 723	23 344	15 225	355 556
KwaZulu-Natal	17 583	78 468	53 105	28 997	28 547	14 584	12 077	11 008	256 542
Mpumalanga	11 108	15 743	22 899	12 401	20 996	16 667	14 953	2 722	117 489
Northern Cape	19 884	10 873	16 838	4 808	16 457	14 584	21 649	14 919	120 012
Limpopo	6 666	4 768	2 387	2 600	4 148	2 588	6 056	2 923	32 136
North West	21 287	20 977	18 367	12 944	14 109	13 885	23 784	6 201	131 554
Western Cape	25 321	43 834	34 575	26 916	17 730	16 634	20 500	4 795	190 305
South Africa	**177 611**	**295 811**	**248 391**	**161 572**	**190 643**	**143 281**	**203 588**	**68 613**	**1 489 510**

Source:UNDP, 2003: 34

EMPLOYMENT/UNEMPLOYMENT

The HDR further informs us that data from household surveys in 1995 and 2001, reflected in income quintiles, show that 87% of the bottom 40% of South African households had none or one working family member and relied heavily for their livelihoods on pensions or remittances in 2001. The HDR underlines that this phenomena is most noticeable in African (black) households, where about 45%

of households in the lowest two income quintiles had no income earners in 2001. Further, an additional 45% of African households in the bottom two quintiles relied heavily on one income earner. These facts are indicative of how vulnerable such households are to the loss of an income or pension. The long-term effect of the apartheid legacy seems to continue to mar the labour market, the HDR notes.

It has been suggested by some of the respondents in the focus groups that the government has not done enough to deal with unemployment; as people who are vulnerable to disease, and who therefore require good nutrition, they would consider action on employment as a motivating factor. Available data from the HDR do indicate high levels of unemployment in present-day South Africa.

Table 43. Employment and unemployment (1995-2002)

		Gender		Type of area		Population	
	Total	Male	Female	Urban	Non-urban	African	Other
1995							
Employed, (official, million)	9 186	5 244	3 941	6 047	3 139	5 882	3 303
Unemployed, (official, million)	1 806	781	1 026	1 107	700	1 495	312
Unemployed, (expanded million)	3 799	1 523	2 276	1 961	1 838	3 330	469
Unemployed rate (official) %	16.4	13.0	20.7	15.5	18.2	20.3	8.0
Unemployed rate (expanded) %	29.3	22.5	36.6	24.5	36.9	36.1	12.4
Labour market participation rate (official) %	45.2	51.0	39.8	54.9	34.0	40.8	58.2
Labour market participation rate (expanded) %	53.4	57.3	49.8	61.5	44.1	50.9	60.8
Labour absorption rate %	37.8	44.4	31.5	46.4	27.8	32.5	53.2
2002							
Employed, (official, million)	11 029	6 184	4 841	7 431	3 598	7 239	3 789
Unemployed, (official, million)	4 837	2 259	2 577	3 186	1 652	4 213	624
Unemployed, (expanded million)	7 925	3 423	4 501	4 389	3 536	7 034	891
Unemployed rate (official) %	30.5	26.8	34.7	30.0	31.5	36.8	14.1
Unemployed rate (expanded) %	41.8	35.6	48.2	37.1	49.6	49.3	19.0
Labour market participation rate (official) %	56.7	63.3	50.7	64.8	45.2	53.8	65.8
Labour market participation rate (expanded) %	67.7	72.0	63.8	72.2	61.5	67.1	69.7
Labour absorption rate %·	39.4	46.4	33.1	45.4	31.0	34.0	56.5

Source:UNDP, 2003: 20.

However, the HDR suggests that although the employment/unemployment figures are negative, the context of these figures must be understood. First and foremost, there is an indication that the high rate of unemployment can be attributed to the dependence of a single bread winner. When this individual dies, the family becomes part of the unemployment category. Secondly, it might be inferred that unemployment does not necessarily mean lack of full employment. The employment category does not account for those who are employed in "low quality jobs", and those who have part-time employment (which usually includes women).

It is not certain from this study what course of action failure on the part of government is likely to provoke. However, there are theoretical perspectives and emergent social phenomena that might lend themselves to further analysis as we move into the next section of this report.

STIGMA AND DISCRIMINATION AS POLITICAL AND SOCIAL PROCESSES

There are, for instance, arguments to the effect that unless we understand the political and social dynamic generated by stigma and discrimination our responses to the pandemic will not be effective in the long term. This line of argument is supported by social and political theory which underlines that stigma and discrimination are not isolated phenomena or simply attitudinal expressions by the individual, but are in fact social processes that are manipulated to generate and sustain social control and produce and reproduce social inequality (Parker, 2002).

Parker and Aggleton (2002) consolidate this argument by highlighting concepts of symbolic violence and hegemony[45] – essentially suggesting that societies achieve conformity by distinguishing between those that are "normal" from those that are "different" and that cultures produce these differences to perpetuate social control. HIV/AIDS, they argue, exacerbates the marginalisation of social groups already sidelined within their cultures, such as blacks, women, gay and bisexual communities and injection drug users.

This might be understood in the context of selective HIV testing of certain race or so-called "high risk" groups when they visit clinics or attempt to apply for bank loans, insurance or bonds and employment. The sum effect of this, of course, is that people who are found to be positive will not usually access all the above benefits and are thus marginalised from economic life. A life of poverty and isolation might result, depending on whether one is in a rural or urban environment.

It has been stated in this study and many others before it, that HIV/AIDS increases poverty by claiming the lives of the breadwinners and causes those infected to lose employment and housing tenure. The HDR report re-affirms that household incomes fall due to the loss of wage earners and rising spending, particularly on medical care and funerals. In both Thailand and Tanzania households are reported to spend up to 50% more on funerals than on medical care.

> *Not only do household outputs and incomes decline, but household members, particularly women, have to make hard choices on the allocation of their time between production, meeting household needs, child care and care of the sick. In a recent study of 700 South African households affected by HIV/AIDS, more than half of the affected families did not have enough food to stave off starvation. Two-thirds of the households reported a loss of income as a result of the disease and larger proportions of household income being spent on health care and funerals.*

So, in short, stigmatisation might play a critical function in transforming divergence based on class, race, ethnicity or sexuality into social inequality. It is posited that a process of legitimisation is instituted causing those discriminated against to internalise their secondary status and accept existing social hierarchies that endure beyond a single generation.

RESISTING THE ESTABLISHED ORDER

But while such hegemony serves to constrain the ability of the marginalised to effectively respond, it does not snuff out their desire to do so. Currency for such arguments is sought in the identity theory which suggests that stigmatised people are capable of resisting the forces that discriminate against them; that they generate "resistance identities", utilise them to assume alternate identities, redefine their position in society and seek overall transformation of social structures. Social mobilisation at all levels, including community, national and international spheres, could result.[46]

Bearing this socio-political dimension in mind, we contextualise the analysis of the outcomes of focus group discussions by relating to how the varied threads of opinion from participants resonate with an emerging global, and certainly national, movement around treatment, care and support for PLWHAs.

The emergence of the Treatment Action Campaign and its Pan-African sibling (the Pan-African Treatment Campaign) confirms this thinking and could be a precursor of things to come if urgency in dealing with HIV/AIDS is consigned to the routines of government bureaucracies.

10.4 GENERAL COMMENTS

We conclude, given the extent of the discourse, that people infected with and affected by HIV/AIDS generally still have a desire to participate in politics provided environmental and structural factors are addressed by authorities. The systematic reduction in the extent of stigma and discrimination and the availability of information on treatment, care and support would greatly boost the confidence levels of such people and encourage them to empathise with the rest of society.

It is certain from this discussion that the increasing pressure on grandparents to care and provide for growing numbers of orphaned children is placing a heavy burden on citizens who are already vulnerable. It is also, we hope, underlined that care givers can themselves be positive and therefore face the multiple threat of stigma, discrimination, loss of employment and income.[47]

We emphasise the seriousness of HIV/AIDS and its potential threat to governance processes as it not only dislocates the economic base by decimating productive members of society but, by doing so, it generates further poverty, creating fissures in societies based on new forms of discrimination and stigma. These might have political consequences in the long term if left unattended, judging by the capacity to mobilise across sectors already demonstrated by social movements in South Africa and the continent at large.

Lastly, South Africa has launched what has been touted as the largest treatment programme in the world. Such programmes are complex, requiring well trained personnel, infrastructure and monitoring mechanisms. Experts from the

World Food Programme (WFP) indicate that treatment programmes are most effective if accompanied by food and nutrition strategies, logically the first line of defence, as people with HIV will require medication only once they progress to AIDS. The wider availability of information and services on treatment and nutrition in Africa should in the long run reduce perceptions of HIV/AIDS as "a death sentence", the underlying refrain that seems to generate much of the stigma and discrimination.

We emphasise that societies must not perpetuate 'differences' between people based on colour, creed, ethnicity language or illness ... there are many ways to 'break the back' of this epidemic. The general framework speaks to the need to develop strategic visions that enable us to project future implications rather than pursue parochial approaches that deal only with today.

Chapter 11

Conclusions and Recommendations

This research, we are confident, has helped define some of the parameters in the relationship between HIV/AIDS and democratic governance. What we have discussed, though, is not about equating HIV/AIDS to a vote. Rather, we explicate the extent to which the very strategic institutions that constitute the state or have potential to form the government have been or might be undermined in one way or another by a pandemic of horrendous proportions.

There obviously is more work to be done in unearthing the consequences of HIV/AIDS for political and social processes in South Africa and Africa in general. For its part, IDASA-GAP will continue to extend and share its know-how with the rest of the continent, depending on the availability of funds.

We believe that a collaborative approach among the states of the AU and research institutions will immensely benefit and support the peoples of Africa to "break the back of the pandemic" – to borrow a phrase from the October 2004 ADF in Addis Ababa, Ethiopia.

We have cautioned our readers already about the potency of disease as a potential destabilising factor in politics; the history of Europe and its great plagues speak for themselves. We have illustrated the extent to which the pandemic has interacted with the political institutions and processes of the South African democratic project and we are hopeful that the information tabled before the government will assist it and its agencies to interrogate these new perspectives further and develop appropriate future strategies.

We also hope that such research grounded in the realm of political governance will be taken on board by the United Nations Commission on AIDS and Governance in Africa; there is, we emphasise, without doubt a connection between the pandemic and the political domain of governance, which quite obviously conditions economic and social outcomes in any country. That the type of governance we analyse is democratic in character speaks to the general direction that Africa and indeed much of the world has chosen to take in this post-cold war era.

We have illustrated the cost or potential burden to the national treasury of AU member states that apply the Westminster methods of elections and explained the benefits of reform grounded in the non-constituency-based PR systems. We have analysed and reached conclusions on the probable effects of the pandemic on the IEC and its planning for future elections. We have critically analysed public perceptions across the southern African region – the growing public awareness of AIDS as a political problem if we do not act comprehensively; the section on voter mortality has more than provided a rare view into what we believe is the closest approximation of the hand of the pandemic in the electoral process yet made. Indeed, we have provided a window for the world to peer into the complex environment that conditions the interaction between People Living with HIV/AIDS (PLWHAs) and their respective communities.

We emphasise that societies must not perpetuate "differences" between people based on colour, creed, ethnicity language or illness. And that, finally, there are many ways to "break the back" of this epidemic. The general framework speaks to the need to develop strategic visions that enable us to project future implications rather than pursue parochial approaches that deal only with today.

11.1 RECOMMENDATIONS

We underline here that the concept of democratic governance carries much normative weight and potentially can be a powerful advocacy tool for a strong political response against the epidemic. As with all such concepts, however, it runs a risk of becoming meaningless, a mere rhetorical phrase, if it is not used in a critical and politically forthright analytical framework that recognises the many previous governance failures on the continent. Here then are the general recommendations arising from our explorative study:

11.1.1 INSTITUTIONAL/STRUCTURAL REFORM

1. Given that an electoral system is the main instrument for translating votes cast in an election into seats for elected representatives, the impact of HIV/AIDS on the system has a direct bearing on the functioning of the two most important representative institutions, Parliament and local government authorities. Thus, one of the most important ways in which the political ramifications of HIV/AIDS on elections can be unveiled by both the academic and policy communities is to discover direct and/or indirect impact of the epidemic on electoral systems as part of the broader electoral reform agenda.
2. As SADC countries embark upon electoral reforms, issues around HIV/AIDS should be taken on board in the determination of appropriate electoral systems to be adopted. By all indications, both the financial and political costs of the HIV/AIDS pandemic are more onerous in countries that operate the FPTP electoral system than those that operate the PR system. In this regard South Africa is better off retaining its PR model at the national level.
3. Currently legislation does not allow for a special vote for people who are unable to travel to polling stations during local government elections. This is a significant omission that might effectively mean that many people infected with HIV or affected by the epidemic will be disenfranchised during local government elections. It is recommended that the IEC should advocate to the Justice Portfolio Committee in Parliament that the Local Government Municipal Electoral Act, No. 24 of 2000 is amended to create a right to a special votes in local government elections.
4. The IEC should finalise the current skills succession plan to ensure that it will have sufficient skilled staff in strategic positions. It must ensure that HIV/AIDS focal-point people are appointed in all offices or that certain staff take responsibilities for HIV/AIDS activities. Such tasks should be part of their formal job descriptions. In addition, the following is recommended:
   a) In the 2004 review of the HIV/AIDS policy proper cognisance must be taken of some of the key limitations of the current policy, namely it does not have a strong gender focus even though 56% of the IEC staff are female, it doesn't cover temporary staff and it does not deal thoroughly with the right to every staff member to treatment, care and support.

b) Staff "buy-in" to the policy and programme must be enhanced by developing a series of seminars and workshops on the impact of HIV/AIDS on the IEC and its staff.
c) The current HIV/AIDS prevention and care programme must be developed through the allocation of additional resources to provincial offices. Current voluntary counselling and testing and stigma programmes must be enhanced.

5. Political parties should consider institutionalising a strong response to the epidemic within its own party structures and membership. The need for democratic governance on HIV/AIDS does not apply only to governments and states, but also to the political parties that through their actions set the norms for what should be an effective government policy and a humane and tolerant attitude in society.

11.1.2 PUBLIC OPINION AND PARTICIPATION

6. The urgency with which HIV/AIDS is addressed through policy by governments and the emphasis it is given by international agencies is not reflected in the most current (from 2002) and comprehensive opinion surveys from sub-Saharan Africa. It is not clear yet how this should be understood and more research is needed. The fact that no obvious political momentum is stirred by issues relating to HIV/AIDS among the electorates in the region does not, however, necessarily imply a lack of concern. Politicians should engage with communities to mobilise a political awareness that can be channelled constructively as part of an overall response to the epidemic.
7. Our results from testing the problematic hypothesis that those directly infected with or affected by the epidemic are more likely not to participate in the electoral process were confirmed, with two exceptions. The lack of data at appropriate levels of analysis, however, generate results that are inherently unstable and thus offer no solid base for political action. Governments and electoral commissions in southern Africa are called upon to assist with the necessary data to enable research with a regional scope that can produce more authoritative results.
8. Our analysis of the mortality profiles among the South African electorate, on the basis of data from the voters' roll, generated information that amounts to the veritable "smoking gun" of AIDS-related mortality. These results should mobilise additional energy for the political response to the epidemic at local, provincial and national levels of government. The information should be discussed further by local communities with local authorities to stem an increase in deaths that in some places is alarmingly high.

11.1.3 Strategic interventions

9. Formation of bi-partisan coalitions. It is recommended that there be greater involvement of political leaders – Members of Parliament and councillors in particular – in public education campaigns to reduce stigma and discrimination; possibly one of the most compelling factors that could impact on voter turnout and registration. This might require the establishment of a strategic bi-partisan extra-parliamentary body that involves all the elected national representatives. Tanzania, for instance, has established the Tanzania Parliamentarians AIDS Coalition (Tapac) the membership of which is open to former and serving MPs from all parties. As Tapac is an NGO and therefore not an integral part of the parliamentary system, it has served to empower MPs, enabled interaction with constituencies and AIDS bodies and continued to improve their advocacy role to enable strong leadership at parliamentary level while maintaining HIV/AIDS on the agenda in parliamentary committees. As nearly all MPs are members of Tapac this set-up provides a good example of a practical way of de-politicising HIV/AIDS, while dealing with issues such as stigma and discrimination.
10. Use of traditional governance systems. It is recommended further that greater emphasis be placed by state and non-state actors in the area of HIV/AIDS on empowering traditional leaders to assist in redressing the problems of stigma and discrimination in rural enclaves to allow for greater participation of PLWHAs in political, social and economic life. The role of traditional leaders in public education and their influence thereof is underlined by respondents in this study who view them as some of the key change agents in dealing with stigma and discrimination in their respective communities. The potential of traditional governance systems to enhance service delivery and ensure that rural populations are not marginalised from development was also underlined and acknowledged by the ADF 1V co-hosted at Addis Ababa, Ethiopia, by the Economic Commission for Africa, the African Union and the African Development Bank in October 2004. Respondents in this study also confirm the critical role played by traditional leaders in sensitising communities on various issues. The use of kingships, councillors and religious leaders through community radio networks and public forums is highly recommended because of the high degree of esteem they seem to command, particularly in rural settings.
11. HIV/AIDS in voter and civic education. It is imperative that the IEC builds HIV/AIDS awareness into its voter education programmes to assist in reducing the extent of HIV/AIDS stigma and discrimination inherent in communities. Establishing linkages with HIV/AIDS service providers and civic education groups should help to develop context-specific approaches to deal with misconceptions about HIV/AIDS and possibly improve or sustain high participation levels. Apart from emphasising all aspects of HIV/AIDS, including prevention, treatment and nutrition, there should be emphasis on the human/political rights of all individuals in the IEC's and civic groups' public communication programmes.

12. We note that South Africa has launched possibly the largest treatment programme in the world. Although the mechanics of it are yet to be lubricated, we see potential in this programme to contribute significantly to efforts to reduce HIV/AIDS-related stigma and discrimination. The sooner the pandemic is seen less as "a death sentence" than a chronic illness, the better for the communities that constantly ostracise PLWHAS for fear of contagion.
13. Monitoring PLWHA participation rates. It is recommended further that election monitoring and observation projects build into their programmes mechanisms for gauging the participation of the marginalised in political processes, in this regard people living with, and stigmatised by, HIV/AIDS. With the increasing number of infections and the likely rise in the extent of orphaning, regular and full participation by the infected and affected might have implications for future political outcomes. Birth registration of orphans is a matter for political representatives to take on board also to ensure that they do not grow into an adulthood that casts doubt on their parentage and therefore their belonging to greater society.
14. We note that the special vote is potentially an effective mechanism for increasing participation in electoral processes. However, it is recommended that specific details on people afflicted by chronic illnesses and those infected with and affected by life-threatening diseases such as HIV/AIDS needs to be included in voter campaign messages to generate higher turnouts. For countries on the African continent that might have problems with managing a special vote facility, exploring possibilities of introducing or extending mobile voting also might be helpful.
15. Adequate logistical arrangements. It might be necessary for South Africa, and certainly member states of the AU, to reassess the structural aspects of the electoral process. We recommend that where necessary polling stations and transport facilities be placed within reasonable reach of all people to facilitate greater participation of citizens, in particular people who are ill with diseases such as HIV/AIDS. Availability of functional ablution facilities within the vicinity of the stations should be an added consideration.

Appendices

Appendix A

"Sad electoral roll deletions," *Natal Witness* 13 April 2004

We have now had 10 years of democracy behind us and we can all judge what has been achieved by those parties in power. The sadness for me has been the increasing number of deaths I have had to record in my "tidying up" of the voter's roll which we use in our election monitoring.

One of the tasks we have done in order to remove the names of those who have died since the voter's roll was last corrected. Unless one is completely insensitive, one can't but help notice the ages of those who have died. Just look at the first two numbers of the person's ID and it will tell you the year they were born in. When you delete an entry for someone with an ID starting 15 or 25, one can be philosophical and say they have had a good innings. But when one deletes IDs starting with the numbers 84 or even 74, then one realises that these South Africans died in their 20s and 30s. The names of the youngsters in the eThekwini area are predominantly Zulu and Xhosa.

The "deceased lists" do not indicate the causes of the death, so one doesn't know for certain whether these young people have died from an HIV/AIDS-related complications. Our president has said he knows no-one with AIDS so you can bet he has never had to do this job. It is really depressing.

Please go out and vote. Do so for all those young South Africans who didn't live long enough to cast their own democratic votes.

GDA PULLMAN
Tongaat
(e-mail, shortened)

APPENDIX B

Table 44. Change (in percent) in numbers of registered voters between 1999 and 2003, per age, gender and province

		Age cohort				
Province	Gender	18-19	20-29	30-39	40-49	50 +
Eastern Cape	Women	-52.7	2.1	13.8	26.8	22.7
	Men	-52.1	7.7	15.0	20.8	24.6
Free State	Women	-47.6	-17.4	6.9	16.8	20.7
	Men	-52.9	-15.4	3.2	16.1	23.3
Gauteng	Women	-55.3	-22.0	9.7	21.4	27..8
	Men	-59.3	-26.0	12.1	18.2	31.3
KwaZulu-Natal	Women	-53.7	-14.2	10.6	18.8	20.4
	Men	-58.6	-11.1	14.0	12.4	24.9
Mpumalanga	Women	-32.8	-8.1	13.1	18.9	23.6
	Men	-48.0	-8.3	9.3	16.0	27.9
Northern Cape	Women	-45.1	-3.1	16.5	22.9	22.4
	Men	-51.8	-3.3	18.2	20.5	22.0
Limpopo	Women	-25.8	8.8	16.7	26.1	21.2
	Men	-42.4	12.6	20.8	19.0	26.3
North-West	Women	-45.9	-7.4	12.8	25.6	23.4
	Men	-51.2	-9.4	8.7	22.2	26.3
Western Cape	Women	-65.5	-14.0	21.6	27.7	28.4
	Men	-69.8	-16.2	21.3	25.2	27.7
National	**Women**	**-49.0**	**-10.5**	**12.7**	**22.5**	**23.5**
	Men	**-54.7**	**-11.2**	**13.3**	**18.3**	**26.8**

Source: IEC (2004). Calculations by authors.

APPENDIX C

Table 45. Absolute numbers of deaths, by age, sex and province, for 1999 and 2003

		Age cohort									
		18-19		20-29		30-39		40-49		50 +	
Province	Gender	1999	2003	1999	2003	1999	2003	1999	2003	1999	2003
Eastern Cape	Women	72	20	1.340	2.998	1.628	4.263	1.517	3.172	10.335	16.818
	Men	108	16	1.365	2.043	2.127	3.560	2.398	3.938	11.028	15.322
Free State	Women	48	6	1.323	1.909	1.757	3.889	1.225	2.502	4.536	6.756
	Men	37	4	957	1.199	2.064	3.542	2.075	3..383	5.068	6.885
Gauteng	Women	71	11	2.562	4.188	3.527	9.030	2.722	6.009	9.490	15.227
	Men	153	8	3.376	3.645	5.421	10.524	4.882	8.642	11.758	17.470
KwaZulu-Natal	Women	112	21	3.502	6.411	3.986	11.065	2.498	5.960	12.031	20.890
	Men	146	21	3.416	4.487	5.242	9.738	4.761	7.802	12.778	18.358
Mpumalanga	Women	43	6	1.001	2.127	1.170	3.439	934	2.137	4.060	6.733
	Men	55	8	972	1.356	1.596	3.132	1.568	2.936	4.805	6.934
Western Cape	Women	17	4	255	386	373	731	392	562	1.589	2.341
	Men	22	4	300	339	487	776	529	808	2.129	2.740
Limpopo	Women	31	8	679	1.421	810	2.461	758	1.704	5.451	8.818
	Men	62	8	585	878	915	1.778	1.135	1.844	5..534	7.487
North-West	Women	30	7	965	1.710	1.211	3.120	974	1.945	4.277	6.619
	Men	34	4	843	1.054	1.528	2.875	1.497	2.840	5.249	7.221
Western Cape	Women	31	4	549	891	758	1.454	729	1.335	4.727	7.823
	Men	80	8	1.098	1.035	1.351	1.998	1.364	2.063	6.206	8.882
National	**Women**	**455**	**87**	**12.176**	**22.041**	**15.220**	**39.452**	**11.749**	**25.326**	**56.879**	**91.985**
	Men	**697**	**81**	**12.912**	**16.036**	**20.731**	**37.923**	**20.209**	**34.256**	**64.555**	**91.299**

Source: IEC (2004). Calculations by authors.

APPENDIX D

THE GOVERNMENT NOTES IDASA STUDY ON HIV AND AIDS AND GOVERNANCE

Government has noted the release by IDASA of their report "HIV/AIDS and Democratic Governance in South Africa". It welcomes the dedication of research effort to issues of public importance and notes the practical nature of the recommendations being made to enhance participation in the electoral process.

At the same time caution needs to be exercised with regard to a number of aspects of the report and it is hoped that media and others will take note of the many caveats and qualifications contained in the report itself, so that the important issues raised are not obscured by sensational responses.

In assessing the implications of the report a number of considerations should be borne in mind.

In assuring the integrity of our institutions and systems there is a myriad of social dynamics that require ongoing attention and we should ensure that all elements of policy - social, economic, and those pertaining to governance as well as safety and security - are worked on taking into account major demographic realities.

These realities include: migration, population growth rate and trends in fertility, changes in household size, and changes in the structure of the economy. AIDS is one such matter, and a very critical one at that, and we welcome the research on this specific dynamic.

The proposal by IDASA that there should be consideration of the findings with regard to HIV and AIDS in electoral planning and other election-related decisions is appreciated. In the same measure, the impact of the other dynamics, such as the ones outlined above, should be factored into such planning.

The same challenge applies to promoting the participation of citizens in the electoral process: the need to take account of the conditions as well as the rights of people living with HIV, generally people with disability, and workers including in particular farm workers. Further, the current under-representation, proportionally, of young people on the electoral roll constitutes another critical challenge for our democratic system.

In other words, electoral planning should seek to incorporate all dimensions of the challenges we face.

The report brings to light interesting data and correctly reminds us that HIV and AIDS affect all sectors of the population. However, by positing worst-case scenarios and projections it then makes the exaggerated conclusion that democracy in South Africa is in danger, that there is a major political risk on the horizon. The report does not bring evidence that the trend in the pandemic has had a fundamental impact on the integrity of political systems anywhere in Southern Africa, including, say Botswana which is supposed to have the highest rate of infection, beyond suggesting that this may have been the case. Related to this is the fact that the populations of countries such as Botswana and Uganda have been growing at the rate of about 2% per annum during the 1990s.

While there is consensus that trends in mortality statistics are reflecting the impact of AIDS in particular amongst young people, the projections cited (from the UNDP and others) regarding population growth and life expectancy are not substantiated and do not appear to be consistent with population growth in our country and other Southern African countries at various stages of the pandemic.

Such worst-case scenarios with the most negative assumptions serve to heighten a sense of crisis. And in discounting the impact of programmes to counter HIV and AIDS, including levels of awareness, reduction in incidence among the youth, impact of treatment programme, the impact of anti-stigma campaigns, the report may serve its purpose in alerting all of society to an issue that requires attention; but it is less valuable in the detail, as a guide to action.

For further information please contact
Dr Lindi Makhubalo
Phone: 012 3210775 or 082 8089853

Issued by Government Communication and Information System (GCIS)

25 November 2004

REFERENCES

LITERATURE

Arndt, C., Lewis, J., 2000. 'The Macro Implications of HIV/AIDS in South Africa: a Preliminary Assessment', *South African Journal of Economics*, August.

Asmal, K. and de Ville, J. 1994. 'An Electoral System for South Africa,' in Steytler, N., Murphy, J., de Vos, P. and Rwelamira, M. (eds.) *Free and Fair Elections*, Kenwyn: Juta & Co, Ltd.

Barrett Grant, CJ., Strode, A. and Smart, R. 2001. *HIV/AIDS in the Workplace: A Guide for Government Departments*. Pretoria: Department of Public Service and Administration.

Baylies, C. and Bujra. J. 1997. 'Social Science Research on AIDS in Africa: Questions of Content,

Bourne, D. 2003. 'Wither the AIDS Epidemic – or lies, damned lies and statistics?' Editorial in *South African Medical Journal* 93 (12): 916.

Bradshaw, D., Laubscher, R., Dorrington, R., Bourne, D., Timaeus, I. 2004. 'Unabated Rise in Number of Adult Deaths in South Africa', *South African Medical Journal*, April.

Bratton, M. and van de Walle, N. 1997. *Democratic Experiments in Africa: Regime Transitions in Comparative Perspective*. Cambridge: Cambridge University Press.

Bray, Rachel. 2003. 'Predicting the Social Consequences of Orphanhood in South Africa'. CSSR Working Paper No. 29, Centre for Social Science Research, University of Cape Town, Cape Town.

Butler, A. 2004. *Contemporary South Africa*. Hampshire: Palgrave Macmillan.

Campbell, Catherine. 2003. 'Letting them Die': How HIV/AIDS Prevention Programmes Often Fail. Cape Town: Double Storey.

Cherry, J. 2004. 'Elections 2004: the Party Lists and Issues of Identity,' *Electionsynopsis*, 1 (3): 6-9.

Chirambo, K., and Caesar, M. (eds.) 2003. *AIDS and Governance in Southern Africa: Emerging Theories and Perspectives*. Pretoria: Idasa.

De Waal, Alex. 2003. 'How Will HIV/AIDS Transform African Governance?' *African Affairs* (102): 1-23.

De Waal, J., Currie, I. and Erasmus, G. 2001. *The Bill of Rights Handbook*. Cape Town: Juta Publishers.

De Ville, J. 1996. 'Proportional Representation: Formulae for the Translation of Votes into Seats,' in De Ville, J. and Steytler, N. (eds.) *Voting in 1999: Choosing an Electoral System*, 19-27.

De Ville, J. and Steytler, N. (eds.) 1996. *Voting in 1999: Choosing an Electoral System*. Durban: Butterworths.

Dorrington, R., Bourne, D., Bradshaw, D., Laubscher, R., Timæus, I.M. 2001. *The Impact of HIV/AIDS on Adult Mortality in South Africa*. Medical Research Council Technical Report, Burden of Disease Unit. Cape Town: MRC.

Dorrington, R., Bradshaw, D. and Budlender, D. 2002. *HIV/AIDS Profile in the Provinces of South Africa: Indicators for 2002*. Centre for Actuarial Research,

Medical Research Council and the Actuarial Society of South Africa: Cape Town.

Dorrington, R., Bradshaw, D., Johnson, L. and Budlender D. 2004. *The Demographic Impact of HIV/AIDS in South Africa: National Indicators for 2004*. Cape Town: Centre for Actuarial Research, South African Medical Research Council and Actuarial Society of South Africa.

Dwivedi, D. 2002. 'On Common Good and Good Governance: An Alternative Approach,' in Olowu, D. and Sako, S. (eds.) 2002. *Better Governance and Public Policy: Capacity Building and Democratic Renewal in Africa*. Bloomfield: Kumarian Press.

EISA Election Observer Mission Report. 2004. *South Africa National and Provincial Elections 12-14 April 2004*. Electoral Institute of Southern Africa

Elbe, Stefan. 2002. 'HIV/AIDS and the Changing Landscape of War in Africa,' *International Security* 27 (2):159-177.

Elklit, J. 2002. 'Lesotho 2002: Africa's First MMP Elections,' *Journal of African Elections* 1 (2): 1-10.

Epstein, Steven. 1996. *Impure Science: AIDS, Activism and the Politics of Knowledge*. Berkeley: University of California Press.

Evian, Clive. 2003. *Primary HIV/AIDS Care*. 4th ed. Durban: Jacana Media.

Fortin, Alfred J. 1990. 'AIDS, Development, and the Limitation of the African State,' in Misztal, B.A. and Moss, D. (eds.) *Action on Aids: National Policies in Comparative Perspective*. New York: Greenwood Press.

Fox, R. and Southall, R. 2003. 'Adapting to Electoral System Change: Voters in Lesotho, 2002,' *Journal of African Elections*, 2 (2), December, 86-96.

Fredland, Richard. 1998. 'AIDS and Development: An Inverse Correlation?' *Journal of Modern African Studies* 36 (4):547-568.

Fredriksson & Kanabus (eds.) 2004. HIV & AIDS Stigma and Discrimination: Attitudes towards HIV and AIDS; http://www.avert.org/aidstigma.htm

Fukuda-Parr, S., Ponzio, R. 2002. 'Governance: Past, Present, Future: Setting the Governance Agenda for the Millennium Declaration,' available at www.undp.org. Geneva: UNDP.

Harris, P. and Reilly, B. (eds.) 1998. *Democracy in Deep-Rooted Conflict: Options for Negotiators*. IDEA Handbook Series, Stockholm: IDEA.

Heywood, Mark. 2000. 'HIV and AIDS: From the Perspective of Human Rights and Legal Protection,' in Sisask, A (ed.) *One Step Further: Response to HIV/AIDS*. Stockholm: Sida.

Heywood, M. 2000. In Jennings R. et al, 2002. *Discrimination & HIV/AIDS*; researched and written for the Department of Health.

Hope, Kempe Ronald, (ed.) 1999. *AIDS and Development in Africa: A Social Science Perspective*. Binghampton: The Haworth Press.

Hsu, Lee-Nah. 2004. *Building Dynamic Democratic Governance and HIV/AIDS Resilient Societies*. Geneva: UNAIDS & UNDP.

Hunter, S. 2003. *Who Cares? AIDS in Africa*. New York: Palgrave Macmillan.

Hyden, G. 1992. 'Governance and the Study of Politics,' in Hyden, G. and Bratton, M. (eds.) 1992. *Governance and Politics in Africa*. Boulder: Lynne Rienner. 1-26.

Hyden, G. and Court, J. 2002. 'Comparing Governance Across Countries and Over Time: Conceptual Challenges,' in Olowu, D. and Sako, S. (eds.) *Better Governance and Public Policy: Capacity Building and Democratic Renewal in Africa*. Bloomfield: Kumarian Press.

Jennings R. et al (2002): *Discrimination and HIV/AIDS: S&T/ALP Research into the Nature and extent of HIV/AIDS discrimination*. Department of Health South Africa.

Jennings R. et al. 2002. *Discrimination & HIV/AIDS*. Researched and written for the Department of Health, South Africa.

Karume, S. 2004. 'Party Systems in the SADC Region: In Defence of the Dominant Party System,' EISA Occasional Papers Series No.16, January.

Kauffman, Kyle D. 2004. 'Why is South Africa the HIV Capital of the World? An Institutional Analysis of the Spread of a Virus,' in Kauffman, K. D. and Lindauer, D. L. (eds.) *AIDS and South Africa: The Social Expressions of a Pandemic*. New York: Palgrave Macmillan.

Kelly, K., Parker, W. and Gelb, S. (eds.) 2002. 'HIV/AIDS, Economics and Governance in South Africa: Key Issues in Understanding the Response,' USAID, South Africa, mimeo.

Krennerich, M. and Nohlen, D. 1998. 'Local Electoral Systems: Options for Reform in South Africa,' in Atkinson, D. and Reitzes, M. (eds.) *From a Tier to a Sphere: Local Government in the New South African Constitutional Order*. Sandton: Heinemann.

Lewis, Jeffrey D. 2004. 'Assessing the Demographic and Economic Impact of HIV/AIDS,' in Kauffman, K. D. and Lindauer, D. L. (eds.) *AIDS and South Africa: The Social Expression of a Pandemic*. New York: Palgrave Macmillan.

Lodge, T. 2004. 'The ANC and the Development of Party Politics in Modern South Africa,' *Journal of Modern African Studies*, 42 (2).

Manning R. 2003. 'The Impact of HIV/AIDS on Local-Level Democracy: A Case Study of the eThekwini Municipality, KwaZulu Natal, South Africa,' CSSR Working Paper No. 35.

Matlosa, K. 2003a. 'Electoral System Reform, Democracy and Stability in the SADC region: A Comparative Analysis,' Electoral Institute of Southern Africa (EISA) Research Report No. 1.

Matlosa, K. 2003b. 'Survey of Electoral Systems and Reform Imperatives in the SADC region,' Electoral Institute of Southern Africa (EISA), Occasional Paper No. 12.

Mattes R, *et al.* 2000. 'Views of Democracy in South Africa and the Region: Trends and Comparisons,' Idasa/CDD/UM.

Mattes, R. 2003. 'Healthy Democracies? The Potential Impact of AIDS on Democracy in Southern Africa,' Institute for Security Studies, Paper 71, April.

Mattes, R. 2004. 'Public Opinion and HIV/AIDS: Facing Up to the Future?' Afrobarometer Briefing Paper, No. 12, April, available at www.afrobarometer.org.

Mbali, Mandisa. 2004. 'HIV/AIDS Policy-Making in Post-Apartheid South Africa,' in Daniel, D., Habib, A. and Southall, R. (eds.) *State of the Nation: South Africa 2003-2004*. Pretoria: HSRC Press.

Morna, C. 2004. *Ringing up the Changes: Gender in Southern Africa Politics.* Johannesburg: Gender Links.

Nattrass, N. 2004. *The Moral Economy of AIDS in South Africa.* Cambridge: Cambridge University Press.

Ngwembe N. 2003. 'Southern African Development Community Electoral Commissions' Forum: The Role of SADC-ECF in Mitigating the Impact of HIV and AIDS on Elections and Electoral Processes,' in Chirambo K. and Caesar M. (eds.) *AIDS and Governance in Southern Africa: Emerging Theories and Perspectives.* Pretoria: Idasa.

Nohlen, D. 1984. *Elections and Electoral Systems.* Bonn: Friederich-Ebert-Stiftung.

Norris, P. 2002. *Democratic Phoenix: Reinventing Political Activism.* Cambridge: Cambridge University Press.

Olaleye, W. 2003. 'Impact of AIDS on Participatory Democracy: Elections, Electorate and Electoral Systems,' in Chirambo, K. and Caesar, M. (eds.) *AIDS and Governance in Southern Africa Emerging Theories and Perspectives.* Pretoria: Idasa.

Olowu, D., Sako, S. 2002. (eds.) *Better Governance and Public Policy: Capacity Building and Democratic Renewal in Africa.* Bloomfield: Kumarian Press.

Ostergard, Robert L Jr. 2002. 'Politics in the Hot Zone: AIDS and National Security in Africa,' *Third World Quarterly* 23 (2):333-350.

Panos/Unicef. 2004. Stigma, HIV/AIDS and Prevention of Mother-to Child Transmission: A pilot study in Zambia, India, Ukraine and Burkina Faso.

Parker R. and Aggleton P. 2002. *HIV/AIDS Related Stigma and Discrimination.* Population Council Inc.

Reynolds, A. (ed.) 1994. *Election '94 South Africa: The Campaigns, Results and Future Prospects.* Cape Town: David Philip.

Reynolds, A. (ed.) 1999. *Election '99 South Africa: From Mandela to Mbeki.* Cape Town: David Philip.

Reynolds, A. and Reilly, B. 2002. 'The International Idea Handbook of Electoral System Design,' Stockholm.

Richter, L., Manegold, J., Pather, R. 2004. *Family and Community Interventions for Children Affected by AIDS.* Cape Town: HSRC.

Sachs, M. 2004. 'Voting Patterns in the 1999 and 2004 Elections Compared', *Electionsynopsis* 1 (4) 2004: 8-12.

Schönteich, Martin and Pharaoh Robyn. 2003. *AIDS, Security and Governance in Southern Africa: Exploring the Impact.* Pretoria: Institute for Security Studies.

Schoofs, Mark. 2000. 'Debating the Obvious: Inside the South African Government's Controversial AIDS Panel,' *Village Voice* July 5 - 11, 2000.

Shilts, R. 1987. *And the Band Played On: Politics, People and the AIDS Epidemic.* New York: Penguin Books.

Shisana, Olive. (ed.) 2002. *Nelson Mandela/HSRC Study of HIV/AIDS: South African National HIV Prevalence, Behavioural Risks and Mass Media.* Cape Town: Human Sciences Research Council, Medical Research Council, Centre for AIDS Development Research and Evaluation, Agence Nationale de Recherches sur le Sida (ANRS).

Shisana, O., Zungu-Dirwayi, N. 2003. 'Government's Changing Responses to

HIV/AIDS', in Everatt d. and Mphai, V. (eds.) *The Real State of the Nation: South Africa After 1990*. Johannesburg: Interfund.

Sisk, T. and Reynolds, A. (eds.) 1998. *Elections and Conflict Management in Africa*. Washington D.C:, United States Institute of Peace.

Smart, R. 1999. 'HIV/AIDS in the Workplace: Principles, Planning, Policy, Programmes and Project Participation,' *AIDS Analysis Africa*, 10 (1) 5.

Southall, R., Mattes, R. 2002. 'Popular Attitudes Towards the South African Electoral System'. CSSR Working Paper, No. 16, November 2002. Centre for Social Science Research, University of Cape Town.

Southall, R. 2004. 'Containing accountability,' *Electionsynoposis*, 1 (1): 6-8.

Sparks, A. 2003. *Beyond the Miracle: Inside the New South Africa*. Johannesburg: Jonathan Ball Publishers.

Strode, A. and Barret Grant, K. 2004. *Understanding the Institutional Dynamics of South Africa's Response to the HIV/AIDS Pandemic*. Cape Town. IDASA.

Van de Walle, N. 2001. *African Economies and the Politics of Permanent Crisis, 1979-1999*. Cambridge: Cambridge University Press.

Van der Vliet, Virginia. 2004. 'South Africa Divided Against AIDS: A Crisis of Leadership,' in Kauffman K. D. and Lindauer, D. L. (eds.) *AIDS and South Africa: The Social Expression of a Pandemic*. New York: Palgrave Macmillan.

Whiteside, Alan. 2000. 'AIDS and the Private Sector,' *AIDS Analysis Africa*, 10, 5.

Whiteside, A. 2002. 'Poverty and HIV/AIDS in Africa,' *Third World Quarterly* 23 (2):313-332.

Whiteside, A, and Barnett, T. 2002. *AIDS in the Twenty-First Century: Disease and Globalization*. Basingstoke: Palgrave MacMillan.

Whiteside, A., Mattes, R., Willan, S. and Manning, R. 2002. 'Examining HIV/AIDS in Southern Africa Through the Eyes of Ordinary Southern Africans'. *Afrobarometer Paper*, No. 12, August 2002.

Whiteside, A. and Sunter, C. 2000. *AIDS: The Challenge for South Africa*. Cape Town: Human & Rousseau and Tafelberg Publishers.

Willan, Samantha. 2000. 'Will HIV/AIDS Undermine Democracy in South Africa?' *AIDS Analysis Africa* 11 (1):14.

Willan, Samantha. 2004. 'Briefing: Recent Changes in the South African Government's HIV/AIDS Policy and its Implementation'. *African Affairs* 103:109-117.

Youde, J. Forthcoming. 'HIV/AIDS and Democratic Legitimacy and Stability in Africa,' in Ostergaard, R. Jr. (ed.) *HIV/AIDS and the Threat to National and International Security*. Hampshire: Palgrave Macmillan.

ELECTION MANIFESTOS AND POLICY STATEMENTS

African Christian Democratic Party: *Election Manifesto 2004*.

African National Congress: *Election Manifesto 2004: A People's Contract to Create Work and Fight Poverty*.

Azanian Peoples' Organisation: *Azanian Peoples' Organisation Policy Positions.*

Democratic Alliance: *Election Manifesto: A better South Africa; Solutions that Work: the DA's Solutions for HIV/AIDS; Election Manifesto 2004: A Programme of Hope.*

Freedom Front: *Election Manifesto 2004.*

Independent Democrats: *Election 2004 Manifesto: Bridging the Divides – Uniting South Africa behind a Common Vision; Health Policy of the Independent Democrats.*

Inkatha Freedom Party: *Election Manifesto 2004: Real Development Now: Let's Make a Difference – Together; IFP AIDS Manifesto: an African and Immediate Response.*

New National Party: *Election Manifesto Nationally; Election Manifesto Western Cape: Cape Plan 2010 HIV and AIDS; Latest Developments on Comprehensive Treatment Plan. 19 November 2003; NNP's HIV/AIDS Perspective: statement by Dr. Kobus Gous, NNP Spokesperson on Health, 13 February 2003.*

Pan African Congress of Azania: *Election Manifesto 2004.*

United Christian Democratic Party: *Election Manifesto: Ready to Govern Where Others Have Failed.*

United Democratic Movement: *Election Manifesto 2004; UDM Health Policy Proposals.*

OFFICIAL SOURCES

August and Another v Electoral Commission and Others (1999 (3) SA 1 (CC))

Certification of the Constitution of the Republic of South Africa (10) BCLR 1253 (CC)

Constitution of the Republic of South Africa Act No. 108 of 1996

Department of Health. 2003. *National HIV and Syphilis Antenatal Sero-Prevalence Survey in South Africa. Summary Report.* Pretoria.

Department of Public Services and Administration. 2000. *Impact and Action Report: Impact of HIV/AIDS on the Public Service.* November 2000. Pretoria

Economic Commission for Africa. 2004. *Striving for Good Governance in Africa: Synopsis of the 2005 African Governance Report Prepared for the African Development Forum IV.* Economic Commission for Africa.

EISA Election Observer Mission Report. South Africa National and Provincial Elections 12-14 April 2004. ISBN: 1-91981461-2. Electoral Institute of Southern Africa.

Electoral Commission Act, No. 51 of 1996

Electoral Commission of Southern Africa (February 2004) *Election Update*, No. 1.

Independent Electoral Commission. 1994. *Report on the National and Provincial Elections, April 1994.*

Independent Electoral Commission. 1999. *Report on the National and Provincial Elections, 2 June 1999.*

Independent Electoral Commission Act, No. 150 of 1993.

Independent Electoral Commission (a) Fact sheet 'Vision & Mission,' available http://www.elections.org.za/Vision.asp on 16 February 2004.
Independent Electoral Commission (b) Frequently Asked Questions, available at http://www.elections.org.za/FAQ.asp 15 January 2004.
Independent Electoral Commission (c) Fact sheet 'Why and How Do I Register?' available at http://www.elections.org.za/Vision.asp 16 February 2004.
Independent Electoral Commission (d) Fact sheet 'Commissioners' available at http://www.elections.org.za/commissioners.asp 20 .January 2004.
Local Government Municipal Structures Act, 1998.
Local Government Municipal Electoral Act, No. 27 of 2000.
Minister of Home Affairs v NICRO and Others CCT $^{3}/_{4}$.
New National Party of South Africa v Government of the RSA (1999 (3) SA 191 (CC)).
Report of the Electoral Task Team, 2002:3.
SADC Principles and Guidelines governing democratic elections, 2004.
South African Government. 2003. *Towards a Ten Year Review*. Pretoria.
Statistics SA. 2001. *Advanced release of recorded deaths 1997-2000. Statistical release P0309.1 Statistics South Africa, Pretoria, December 2001.*
Statistics SA. 2004. *Mid-year population estimates, South Africa 2004*. Statistical release P0302. Pretoria: Statistics South Africa.
UNAIDS. 2002. *Report on the Global HIV/AIDS Epidemic, July*.
UNAIDS. 2003. *Epidemiological Update*. Geneva: UNAIDS.
UNAIDS. 2004. *Report on the Global AIDS Epidemic*. Geneva: UNAIDS.
UNDP. 1997. *Reconceptualising Governance: Discussion Paper 2*. UNDP Management Development and Governance Division. New York: UNDP, available at www.undp.org
UNDP. 2002a. *Human Development Report*, Oxford: Oxford University Press.
UNDP. 2002b. *Assessment of UNDP Assistance for a Multi-Sectoral National Response to HIV/AIDS in Tanzania*. Pretoria: UNDP.
UNDP. 2002c. *Deepening Democracy in a Fragmented World*. UNDP Human Development Report 2002, New York, available at www.undp.org
UNDP 2003. *South Africa Human Development Report 2003: The Challenge of Sustainable Development in South Africa: Unlocking People's Creativity*. Geneva: UNDP.
World Bank. 2000. *Intensifying Action Against HIV/AIDS in Africa: Responding to a Development Crisis*. Washington: The World Bank.

INTERVIEWS

DUDLEY, Cherryllyn. Spokesperson on HIV/AIDS for the African Christian Democratic Party. Cape Town, 2004-03-15.
GOUWS, Kobus. Spokesperson on HIV/AIDS for the New National Party. Cape Town, 2004-03-18.
GRAHAM, Paul. Director of IDASA. Pretoria, 2004-08-19.

GREYLING, Lance. Spokesperson on HIV/AIDS for the Independent Democrats. Cape Town, 2004-09-11.
HENDRICKSE, Michael. Senior Manager in the Electoral Democracy, Training and Legal Services Division of the IEC. Pretoria, 2004-06-07.
KARIEM, Saadiq. Secretary of the Health Committee for the African National Congress. Cape Town, 2004-06-04.
MOSERY, Mawetu. Provincial Electoral Officer in KwaZulu-Natal. Durban, 2004-06-03.
MZAIDUME, D. IEC. 2004-08-03.
RABINOWITZ, Ruth. Spokesperson on HIV/AIDS for the Inkatha Freedom Party. Telephonic interview, 2004-04-23.
SAMPSON, C. Provincial Electoral Officer in the Western Cape. 2004-05-28.
WATERS, Mike. Spokesperson on HIV/AIDS for the Democratic Alliance. Cape Town, 2004-02-26.

NEWSPAPER MATERIAL

Business Day, 28 October 2004; 12 November 2004.
Mail & Guardian, 19 to 25 March 2004.
The Star, 26 January 2004.

MISCELLANEOUS

Badcock-Walters P., Desmond C., Wilson D. and Heard W. 2003. Educator Mortality in Service in KwaZulu-Natal, HEARD available at www.heard.org.za
Chirambo K. 2003. 'Impact of HIV/AIDS on Electoral Processes in Southern Africa,' presentation at the UNDP/Idasa Satellite Conference on AIDS and Governance held at the 13th ICASA Conference, Nairobi, September 2003.
Chirambo, K. 2004. 'AIDS and Electoral Democracy: Implications for Participation, Political Stability and Accountability in Southern Africa,' Idasa, mimeo.
Coetzee, Ryan. E-mail communication with PS, policy proposal attached. 19 October 2004.
Fuare, M. and Venter, A. 2003. 'Electoral Reform in South Africa,' University of South Africa/Rand Afrikaans University, South Africa, mimeo.
George, G. 2003. Company Practices on HIV/AIDS in the Durban Metropolitan Area, HEARD, University of Natal.
HIV/AIDS stigma: Making the Connection to Discrimination and Prejudice: www.socialworkers.org
IEC. 2004. Data set from the voters' roll, detailing registered and deceased voters for the five years 1999 to 2003, per gender, per age cohort and per municipality. IEC: Pretoria.

IDASA-GAP. 2003. AIDS and governance in Zambia, research commissioned by IDASA.

IDASA-GAP verbatim transcripts of focus group discussions in KwaMashu, Inanda, Nongoma, (KwaZuluNatal, South Africa). Conducted for IDASA-GAP by Citizen Surveys, 2004

Konrad-Adenauer-Stiftung. 2003. 'Electoral Models for South Africa: Reflections and Options,' Johannesburg, mimeo.

Matlosa, K. 2004. 'Democratic Governance and the Role of Political Parties in Parliament: the Case of Lesotho,' paper prepared for a conference on Government and Opposition-Roles, Rights and Responsibilities, jointly hosted by Commonwealth Parliamentary Association, SADC Parliamentary Forum and FECIV, Maputo, Mozambique, 26-30 January.

Mattes R. et al 2000. *Views of Democracy in South Africa and the Region: Trends and Comparisons*. Idasa/CDD/UM

Mfenyana, S. 2004. Secretary of Parliament. Letter in response to request for information from Dr. P. Strand. Cape Town, 1 April 2004.

National Association of Social Workers. 2002. *Worlds AIDS Day: HIV/AIDS Stigma: Making the Connection to Discrimination and Prejudice; Forcible Segregation of HIV Positive Prisoners in Alabama* www.socialworkers.org

TAPAC. Information on the Tanzania Parliamentarians AIDS Coalition on www.tapac.org accessed on 7 July 2004.

Tapfumaneyi, W. O. 2003. 'Impact of HIV/AIDS on Elections and Electoral Systems in Zambia,' IDASA.

The Encyclopedia of Democracy, 1995. London: Routledge.

UNAIDS fact sheet. http://japan.usembassy.gov/e/p/tp-gi04.html

Wisten, Anne, forthcoming. "Does HIV/AIDS Generate Corruption? Testing a Link Between the Epidemic and Good Governance in Africa,' mini-thesis presented to the Department of Government at Uppsala University, Sweden.

ENDNOTES

1 Our discussion of the epidemic does not claim to be complete or exhaustive, but rather focussed on the particular theme for the report. In most cases the omissions we make on that basis are quite natural and uncontroversial. We do wish to comment briefly on one that could be said to be less obvious. The many children that are orphaned due to AIDS – whether or not they are themselves infected – could and should be analysed also from a governance perspective. The extraordinary hardships that orphans often have to endure will most likely have an adversarial effect on their chances and perhaps inclinations to becoming citizens steeped in a culture of democracy. With no or little parental guidance and support the risk increases that orphans are forced to seek out an existence at the periphery of society and its democratic processes. In other words, unless society mounts a

huge effort to embrace orphans into caring families and communities, the incentives for them to, in turn, take an individual responsibility for participating in the democratic society and its electoral processes are likely to be very weak. See further Richter et al (2004), Bray (2003).

2 Some additional comments on the statistical analyses will be provided in the endnotes in the respective chapters.

3 At the stage of our final editing of the manuscript for this publication, Professor Rob Dorrington and his colleagues published a report based on the ASSA2000 model that estimated the national HIV prevalence in South Africa to 5 million, slightly lower than the 2004 UNAIDS report. For reasons of timing the most recent report from Dorrington et al has not been worked into this document to the extent that it should. However, since the report does not present updated estimates and projections for the different provinces (which would have been useful for our correlation analyses) we will use their previous report (Dorrington 2002) for these purposes.

4 We disregard the higher estimates given by HSRC for women 40-49 years old as these do not correspond to the reporting of the same ages by the DoH, but also because the antenatal clinic data have a weak basis for estimating prevalence in this age cohort.

5 The HDI has a negative correlation with AIDS deaths (Pearson's r = ..36) and with AIDS sickness (Pearson's r = .28). The HPI has a positive correlation with AIDS deaths (Pearson's r = .81) and with AIDS sickness (Pearson's r = .70).

6 It would be expected that HIV estimates correlate negatively with HDI since prevalence should be higher where indicators of development are lower. The correlation with HPI is significant at a .01 level. When plotted, the nine cases are clearly centred on the regression line. The very strong correlations between poverty indicators and the ASSA model are in parts explained by the fact that the model builds on such poverty data in generating its estimates.

7 This section builds mainly on the different contribution in Göran Hyden and Michael Bratton (1992).

8 Economic governance refers to economic policy and political economy in general; administrative governance refers to bureaucratic processes, and systemic governance captures how a political system represents and protects post-modern values such as identity and environment.

9 The Millennium Summit was held at the UN headquarters in New York in September 2000. In his address to the summit the Secretary-General outlined the development goals that subsequently were formulated more precisely in a report presented a year later. The report formulates 8 development goals, sets 18 targets and identifies the 48 indicators by which progress towards meeting the goals will be measured. Goal number 6 is to "combat HIV/AIDS, malaria and other diseases". The target in relation to HIV/AIDS is to "have halted by 2015 and begun to reverse the spread of HIV/AIDS", which will be measured by the three indicators "HIV preva-

lence among 15 to 24 year-old pregnant women; contraceptive prevalence rate, and; number of children orphaned by HIV/AIDS". See further about the Millennium Campaign at www.un.org.

10 See Chirambo K and McCullum H. (2000). Reporting Elections in Southern Africa: A Media Handbook. SARDC/USAID

11 At the time of writing this report, Mrs Priscilla Isaacs was Deputy Director of the Electoral Commission of Zambia and the interview was conducted telephonically

12 While the regulation of public broadcasting in a fair and non-partisan way is very important during the period leading to elections, the structure and mandate of ICASA fall outside the primary scope of this report.

13 According to the IEC its provincial offices had the following number of staff in June 2004: KwaZulu-Natal (13), Gauteng (11), Western Cape (9), Limpopo (10), Eastern Cape (11), Free State (9), Northern Cape (10), North West (10) and Mpumalanga (9).

14 It was noted during an interview with Mr Mosery of the IEC's KwaZulu Natal office that this point was currently the subject of a legal dispute at the Commission on Conciliation, Mediation and Arbitration (CCMA).

15 The other Chapter Nine institutions are the Public Protector, the Human Rights Commission, the Commission for the Promotion and Protection of the Rights of Cultural, Religious and Linguistic Communities, the Commission for Gender Equality and the Auditor General.

16 The right to vote in free and fair elections.

17 These government departments were selected as their staffing profile are in some respects similar to the IEC.

18 The outline is based on Nattrass, 2004; Shisana and Zungu-Dirwayi, 2003; Sparks, 2003; Kauffman, 2004; and van der Vliet, 2004.

19 See list of party electioneering material in the list of references. In order to increase the flow of the text, citations will be taken from one or more of the respective documents detailed here as the different parties are discussed without further notation in the text.

20 A policy accord between the main parties in Botswana has presented the population with a unified political establishment working together against prejudice and for effective implementation of a very ambitious overall response to the epidemic (Tlou, 2004). The parliamentary parties in Tanzania have created the Tanzania Parliamentarians AIDS Coalition (TAPAC). Launched in August 2001 by MPs from different parties, TAPAC seeks to mobilise parliamentarians so they are more effective in implementing various aspects of the national response to the epidemic in their respective constituencies. See www.tapac.org

21 Our various efforts to learn more from the ANC about this survey came to nothing. Saadiq Kariem referred to the survey more generally and was unsure if the results had ever even been reported on in a comprehensive manner within the ANC.

22 Correlations (Pearson's r) were .233 and .252 for 'men' and 'urban' respectively, both at .01 level, and between .097 to .166 for other categories. Only

the black racial group had an 'N' large enough to uphold these statistical analyses, with a correlation of .195.

23 The unstandardised regression coefficients were considerable in all categories – all South Africans .219, black .155, male .270, female ..188, black women .167, urban .289 and rural .115 – and they were all statistically significant at .01 level except for 'rural' which was significant at .05 level.

24 In a factor analysis, the three variables loaded .921 (household member), .713 (self) and .454. We decided to keep all three variables in the scale since a reliability analysis gave Alpha .7280 for the three variables.

25 The degree of activism in civil society was captured in two sets of questions. In the first the respondent was asked whether she is 'not a member', an 'inactive member', an 'active member', or an 'official leader' of four different kinds of civil society organisations (see table 7.4.) – all of which can be said to have a more or less political agenda. In the second set of questions the respondent was asked to say whether during the last year she had done any of the four 'activities' that are listed in table 7.4. The response alternatives were 'no, would never do this', 'no, but would do it if had the chance', 'yes, once or twice', 'yes, several times', and 'yes, often'. The fifth 'activity' in survey – 'used force or violence for a political cause' – has been omitted here since it yielded no statistically significant correlations at all. The response option 'Don't know' (roughly 1 to 4 percent of responses for the different questions) has been recoded as missing value..

26 The question read: 'Overall, how satisfied are you with the way democracy works in South Africa?' The response options were 'South Africa is no democracy', 'not at all satisfied', not very satisfied', fairly satisfied', and 'very satisfied'. 'Don't know' responses had been recoded as missing values.

27 There is an important distinction to be made in relation to VAP. The mere fact of citizenship and being 18 years or more does not qualify a person to participate in the election since the person also need to have the required ID document. The more precise term would therefore be the voting-eligible-population (VEP). Officials at the IEC however told us that the difference between he two terms in the South African context is marginal.

28 When the correlation tests were plotted it was obvious that the Western Cape fell outside of the general picture. Some correlation analyses were therefore conducted without the WC, as reported above.

29 The release of the data was an example of the IEC's commitment to assisting us in our research, as expressed in a letter from the IEC's Chief Electoral Officer, Advocate Pansy Tlakula. Before the material was handed to us its release was also sanctioned by the IEC commissioners.

30 While we argue that the provincial level mortality profiles reflect AIDS mortality in South Africa, we are not making the same general claim for the municipal level profiles. These maps will have to be scrutinised further in order to establish to what extent the variations in mortality are consistent with the HIV/AIDS hypothesis. For instance, while the municipal level maps for the KwaZulu-Natal province suggest no apparent challenge to that hypothesis, it is perhaps more problematic as an explanation to the varia-

tions in the Northern Cape province. Our presentation here makes no claim to explore these issues in full, but describes the variations in mortality profiles on the municipal level that still needs to be explained with greater precision.

31 This analysis can of course be taken much further through regression analyses under different assumptions, explorations that we hope to return to in other publications.

32 The results from a series of partial correlations introduce much complexity into the general picture that we described through the correlations in tables 9.2 and 9.3. In these tests we started by repeating the tests for correlation between the increases in mortality and the various estimates and projections of the epidemic that we did in section 9.3.1, but this time we 'controlled for' the effect of the variations in the HPI. What this means is that we tested the strength and significance of the correlation between the epidemic and mortality in the provinces while making sure that the scale of human poverty in the provinces did not influence that correlation. After that we turned the logic around and tested the correlation between poverty and mortality while controlling, one by one, for the different estimates and projections of the epidemic. The full table of correlation coefficients and their significance are provided in appendix X. Suffice it here to say that the theoretical suggestions that both the epidemic and poverty are valid predictors for the increase in mortality are borne out by our analysis to some extent in the bivariate correlation analyses. How the two variables interact more precisely and what is the strength of their effect we will leave for subsequent analyses to explore further.

33 UNAIDS fact sheet. http://japan.usembassy.gov/e/p/tp-gi04.html

34 In the pilot study in Zambia, it was found that while on the one hand local churches preached morality and compassion for the sick, they viewed HIV/AIDS as a punishment and refused to discuss HIV prevention interventions.

35 See National Association of Social Workers 2002 Worlds AIDS Day: HIV/AIDS Stigma: Making the Connection to Discrimination and Prejudice; *Forcible Segregation of HIV Positive Prisoners in Alabama.* www.socialworkers.org

36 The case of *Hoffman vs SAA*. The Constitutional Court held that SAA unfairly discriminated against Hoffman, who was denied employment after a pre-employment test.

37 A survey in Nigeria among 2 000 physicians, nurses and midwives conducted in 2002 found that one in ten doctors and nurses refused to attend to HIV/AIDS patients or denied them access to treatment. Quoted in Fredriksson & Kanabus, 2004.

38 A recent survey found that the status of 29% of people with HIV/AIDS in India, 38% in Indonesia and 40% in Thailand said their HIV status had been revealed by medical staff.

39 Available on www.unicef.org

40 www.socialworkers.org: HIV/AIDS stigma: Making the Connection to

Discrimination and Prejudice

41 According to the SADC Principles and Guidelines governing democratic elections, 'the SADC Guidelines are not only informed by the SADC legal and policy instruments but also by the major principles and guidelines emanating from the OAU/AU Declaration on the Principles Governing Democratic Elections in Africa – AHG/DECL.1 (XXXVIII) and the AU Guidelines for African Union Electoral Observation and Monitoring Missions – EX/CL/35 (III) Annex II'.

42 There are five major television channels: SABC 1/2/3 and SABC Africa; e-TV, the pay Channels MNET and DSTV which has over 100 satellite channels. There are some 38 commercial radio stations using both local languages and English as a medium of communication; 70 or more community stations; 16 daily newspapers; 25 weeklies, among others.

43 See Afrobarometer study 2002: *Views of Democracy in South Africa and the Region: Trends and Comparisons*. Opinions of ordinary persons sampled in Botswana, Zimbabwe, Zambia, Malawi, Namibia and South Africa place job creation, the economy, education, crime and security, health and poverty among the highest priorities for government to act upon.

44 The HSRC's 2002 joint study with the Nelson Mandela Foundation asserts that while South Africans are generally well exposed to media messages and while radio provides the widest multi-lingual diversity, African languages tend to be marginalised. The study notes that regular exposure to broadcast media is low in rural areas and poorer households. The most pervasive messages on HIV/AIDS related to condom use; other slogans were around fidelity, abstinence, emphasis on religious or cultural values, care provision for people with HIV/AIDS, and rights of people with HIV/AIDS.

45 Ibid., citing Bordieu 1977; 1984; 1977: Symbolic violence is a process where words, images and practices promote the interests of the dominant group and hegemony is achieved through the use of political, social and cultural forces to promote the dominant meanings and values that legitimise unequal structures (Foucault 1977; Gramsci 1970; Williams 1977; Williams 1982).

46 Ibid.

47 UNDP HDR 2003 reports that the number of households whose primary care givers are under the age of 18 years is also increasing. This has the knock-on result of decreasing school attendance and retarding efforts to build human capital. Other social implications include the abandonment and abuse of people living with HIV/AIDS, stigmatisation, poor morale and stress.

ABBREVIATIONS

ANC	African National Congress
AU	African Union
AIDS	Acquired Immune Deficiency Syndrome
ACDP	African Christian Democratic Party
ANC	African National Congress
ANC data	HIV prevalence data from ante-natal clinics
ARV	Anti-Retro Viral treatment
CARE	Centre for Actuarial Research
DA	Democratic Alliance
DoH	Department of Health (South Africa)
EC	Eastern Cape province
EMBs	Electoral Management Bodies
FPTP	First-Past-the-Post electoral system
FS	Free State province
GDP	Gross Domestic Product
GNU	Government of National Unity
GT	Gauteng province
HIV	Human Immuno-deficiency Virus
ICASA	Independent Communication Authority of South Africa
ID	Independent Democrats
IEC	Independent Electoral Commission
IFP	Inkatha Freedom Party
HDI	Human Development Index
HPI	Human Poverty Index
HSRC	Human Sciences Research Council
KZN	KwaZulu-Natal province
L	Limpopo province
MEO	Municipal Electoral Officers
M	Mpumalanga province
MMP	Mixed Member Proportional electoral system

MP	Member of Parliament
MTCT	Mother to Child Transmission
NACOSA	National AIDS Committee of South Africa
NC	Northern Cape province
NNP	New National Party
NW	North-West province
PLWHA	People Living with HIV/AIDS
PR	Proportional Representation electoral system
SADC	Southern African Development Community
SANAC	South African National AIDS Commission
STI	Sexually Transmitted Infection
TAC	Treatment Action Campaign
UDM	United Democratic Movement
UNAIDS	Joint United Nations Programme on AIDS
UNDP	United Nations Development Programme
VAP	Voting Age Population
WC	Western Cape province

www.ingramcontent.com/pod-product-compliance
Ingram Content Group UK Ltd.
Pitfield, Milton Keynes, MK11 3LW, UK
UKHW051452290926
15471UKWH00008B/1162

9 781919 798806